ABC OF CHILD ABUSE

ABC OF CHILD ABUSE

THIRD EDITION

edited by

SIR ROY MEADOW FRCP CH

Professor of Paediatrics and Child Health, St James's University Hospital, Leeds
Inaugural President, Royal College of Paediatrics and Child Health

with contributions by

FRANK BAMFORD, INGRID DAVISON, SYLVIA FRASER, JANE GILMOUR, CHRIS HOBBS,
ALEX LEVIN, BARBARA MITCHELS, RORY NICOL, MICHAEL PRESTON-SHOOT, RAINE ROBERTS,
DAVID SKUSE, NIGEL SPEIGHT

BMJ
Publishing
Group

© BMJ Publishing Group, 1989, 1993, 1997

First printed 1989
Second impression 1991
Second edition 1993
Third edition 1997

British Library Cataloguing Publication Data
A catalogue record for this book is available from the British Library

ISBN 0–7279–1106–6

Typeset by Apek Typesetters Ltd., Nailsea, Bristol
Printed and bound by Craft Print, Singapore

Contents

Contributors

Frank Bamford
Former Reader in Developmental Paediatrics and Consultant Paediatrician
University of Manchester

Ingrid Davison
Consultant in Child and Family Psychiatry
Leicester

Sylvia Fraser
Author and Journalist
Toronto, Canada

Jane Gilmour
Research Psychologist
Institute of Child Health, London

Chris Hobbs
Consultant Community Paediatrician
St James's University Hospital, Leeds

Alex Levin
Assistant Professor
Departments of Ophthalmology and Paediatrics, University of Toronto, Hospital for
Sick Children, Canada

Sir Roy Meadow
Professor of Paediatrics and Child Health
St James's University Hospital, Leeds

Barbara Mitchels
Children Panel Solicitor, Psychotherapist
Norwich

Rory Nicol
Professor of Child Psychiatry
Greenwood Institute of Child Health, Leicester

Michael Preston-Shoot
Professor of Social Work and Social Care
Liverpool John Moore's University

Raine Roberts MBE
Forensic Physician
Greater Manchester Police

David Skuse
Professor of Behavioural Sciences, Institute of Child Health, London
and Honorary Consultant, Department of Psychological Medicine, Hospital for Sick
Children, London

Nigel Speight
Consultant Paediatrician
Dryburn Hospital, Durham

PREFACE

The first edition of the *ABC of Child Abuse* was published in 1989, at a time when sexual abuse was reaching the headlines and the new *Children Act* was just coming into force. This third edition profits from much greater experience of all forms of abuse, as well as of procedures under the 1989 legislation and the impact that those have had on child protection.

For this edition all the chapters have been revised, and in those topics in which there has been the most major change the sections have been rewritten, though the format and layout are similar to previous editions. As is fitting for a subject requiring multidisciplinary collaboration, the authors include paediatric specialists, child psychiatrists, a forensic physician, opththalmologist, psychologist, social scientist, and lawyer.

The book remains primarily a text for doctors about the recognition and diagnosis of child abuse. It emphasises those aspects of the clinical history, examination, and investigation which are useful in deciding whether the child's problems are the result of natural or unnatural (abusive) causes. As always the medical contribution depends not just on doctors but on the nurses and other staff of the health service who deal with children and who may be the first to notice abuse or be informed of it. This book should help them. It will also be helpful to all those concerned with child protection, whether from social services, the police, and legal or teaching professions, in understanding the way that the medical diagnosis is made and the strengths and weaknesses of medical opinions and reports. The book outlines procedures and the respective roles of all who contribute to child protection but does not go into the detail of management.

The level of knowledge is that to which a consultant paediatrician should aspire and, regardless of their particular specialty interest, all consultant paediatricians need to be knowledgeable about child abuse because of its commonness and the diversity of its presentation. For general practitioners, accident and emergency staff, and other medical specialists there should be more than enough information in this book. On the other hand, those consultant paediatricians who spend a major part of their time in child protection work are the people who are most likely to use the references listed as further reading.

The further reading includes several important and authoritative national guidelines which have been published in the past six years. In addition to those national guidelines there are usually good and appropriate local guidelines about procedures to be followed when child abuse is suspected or detected. This book should be used in conjunction with those guidelines.

SIR ROY MEADOW
St James's University Hospital
Leeds

Acknowledgements

I thank paediatricians and other colleagues who have referred complex cases to me and who, by their descriptions, discussion, and insight, have taught me much. I also thank the medical illustration departments at St James's University Hospital, Leeds, Royal Victoria Infirmary, Newcastle, General Hospital, Newcastle, and Dryburn Hospital, Durham, and Dr Myles Clarke for illustrations. The drawing of retinal haemorrhage is reproduced from Ludwig S, Kornberg AE, *Child Abuse, A Medical Reference*. New York: Churchill Livingstone, 1991.

The help and careful work of Mandy Jones is acknowledged with much gratitude.

EPIDEMIOLOGY

Roy Meadow

This week at least four children in Britain will die as a result of abuse or neglect. This year most departments of social services and of child health will be notified of more than 20 times as many cases of suspected child abuse as they were 10 years ago. Although some of the reports will prove to be unfounded, the common experience is that proved cases of child abuse are four or five times as common as they were a decade ago. The names of nearly 35 000 children in England are listed on child protection registers. This poses enormous burdens on staff in the health and social services and raises many problems about the lives and welfare of children in our society. Determining whether there is a true increase of child abuse or whether the figures merely reflect increased awareness rests to some extent on the definition of child abuse.

Definition

A child is considered to be abused if he or she is treated in a way that is unacceptable in a given culture at a given time. The last two clauses are important because not only are children treated differently in different countries but within a country, and even within a city, there are subcultures of behaviour and variations of opinion about what constitutes abuse of children. Moreover,

standards obviously change over the years: corporal punishment has become significantly less acceptable in Britain in the past 10 years. Looking back further there is evidence that the abuse of children by parents was considered to be culturally acceptable in Britain 100 years ago. At the time that Lord Shaftesbury was creating better conditions for children at work he was unwilling to tackle the problem of child abuse at home.

> The evils are enormous and indisputable, but they are so private, internal and domestic a character as to be beyond the reach of legislation and the subject would not, I think, be entertained in either House of Parliament.
> LORD SHAFTESBURY, 1880

In fact the first charter for children appeared in 1889, some 67 years after the introduction of legislation to protect animals.

Types of abuse

Physical abuse (non-accidental injury)—The prototype of physical abuse, "the battered baby", was rediscovered by Henry Kempe of Denver, Colorado, in 1962 and has been well publicised ever since. Physical abuse entails soft tissue injury to the skin, eyes, ears, and internal organs as well as to ligaments and bones. Burns and scalds are included. Most of this abuse is short term and violent, though it

Poisoning

Pinching

Breaking

Epidemiology

Punching

Slapping

Lashing

Raping

Scalding

Burning

may be repetitive. There is, however, a subgroup that entails more long term deliberate injury, including poisoning and suffocation.

Neglect—This is failing to provide the love, care, food, or physical circumstances that will allow a child to grow and develop normally. Or it is exposing a child to any kind of danger.

Sexual abuse—This occurs when dependent, developmentally immature children and adolescents participate in sexual activities that they do not fully comprehend, to which they are unable to give informed consent, and that violate the social taboos of family roles. Such abuse ranges from inappropriate fondling and masturbation to intercourse and buggery. Children may also be forced to participate in producing pornographic photographs and videos, or be victims of extended family network abuse, sex rings, or ritual abuse.

Emotional abuse—This has no generally agreed definition. Some regard a child as abused if he or she has a behavioural disturbance to which the parents fail to respond appropriately in terms of modifying

their behaviour or seeking professional help. Most would consider a child to be emotionally abused, however, if the child's behaviour and emotional development were severely affected by the parents' persistent neglect or rejection. Thus emotional abuse may lead to a failure to thrive and short stature in young children. Other less common forms of emotional abuse include Munchausen syndrome by proxy, in which the parents force the child into a role of inappropriate illness.

Commonly, different types of abuse overlap with each other so a child may be abused in several different ways either at the same time or sequentially.

Clearly, in most forms of abuse the abuser, usually the parent, may harm the child both actively and passively and by acts of both commission and omission. One parent may be active in beating the child, another just as harmful by passively failing to protect a child from the sexual advances of a cohabitant. A parent who passively fails to provide food or love for a child may indulge also in active physical assault.

Starving   Cutting   Buggering

Prevalence

Four per cent of children up to the age of 12 are brought to the notice of professional agencies (social service departments or the National Society for the Prevention of Cruelty to Children) because of suspected abuse. Some of that abuse is not proved and some of it is mild, but a British survey has shown that each year at least one child per 1000 under the age of 4 years suffers severe physical abuse—for example, fractures, brain haemorrhage, severe internal injuries, or mutilation. A minimum mortality is one in 10 000 children; most people concerned with child abuse believe the mortality to be considerably higher as many cases are undetected.

The prevalence of other types of abuse is even more difficult to determine. Much depends on how the abuse is defined and whether minor degrees of abuse are included in a study. This problem is particularly apparent in sexual abuse.

Most adults can remember an unpleasant sexual event or inappropriate approach that was made to them as a child but, if it was merely someone who indulged in indecent exposure on one occasion or fumbled about his or her clothing, may not consider that they have been sexually abused. Most reported instances of sexual abuse do not entail physical contact. Clinical experience suggests that sexual abuse is most damaging when it is repeated, perpetrated by family members, or entails physical contact backed by force or threats.

Many of the recent mass surveys have failed to distinguish between different types of abuse or to deal with the severity or repetition of the abuse. Moreover, the authors sometimes seem to forget the limitations of adults in reporting past sexual experiences, particularly if they are doing so at a time of emotional upset (perhaps

Freud's writings of 90 years ago should be compulsory reading for all research workers). Home Office criminal statistics yield merely a few hundred cases a year of sexual abuse of children and grossly underrepresent the true incidence, tending more to reflect detection skills and prosecution practice. The yearly incidence of sexual abuse in 1995 was 0·75 cases per 1000 children. This figure is based on the number of children entered on to child protection registers because of sexual abuse that year. It reflects the degree of suspicion at that time and the practices of the local authorities keeping the child abuse registers: it does not give any indication of the type or severity of the abuse or the extent of undetected abuse.

Thus, although there is some evidence that there may have been an increase in some forms of child abuse in the past 10 years, the current escalation of reported cases and identified cases is much more a matter of public awareness, better professional recognition, and an unwillingness by society to tolerate the abuse of children.

Although the thresholds for defining child abuse have moved steadily lower, professionals have become more mindful of the potentially damaging effects of over-zealous intervention (three-quarters of partnerships break up within one year of allegations of child abuse). Similarly they are wary of removing children from their families because of uncertainty that the state necessarily is a better parent than an abusing or inadequate biological parent.

Aetiology

Boys and girls are both abused. First born children are more often affected, and within a family it is common for just one of the children to be abused and the others to be free from such abuse. Young children are most at

3

In April 1995, 35 000 children were on child protection registers in England, a rate of 3·2 children per 1000 population below the age of 18 years. Nearly a quarter of the children on the registers were in the care of local authorities, and another 3% were subject to supervision orders. The highest rates for registration are for children under the age of 5 years.

Child protection registers

Main reason for child being on register (1995)

Physical abuse	40%
Neglect	30%
Sexual abuse	24%
Emotional abuse	6%

(Girls accounted for 61% of those registered under sexual abuse and for 47% of those registered under physical abuse.)

risk, partly because they are more vulnerable and partly because they cannot seek help elsewhere. Children under 2 years of age are most at risk from severe physical abuse. Death from abuse is rare after the age of 1 year.

Most abuse is by the child's parents, and it is particularly common for a parent or cohabitant who is living in the home but is not related to the child to be the abuser. Young parents are more likely to abuse than older ones. It is common for both parents to be involved with physical abuse and neglect; sex abuse is more commonly perpetrated by men, whilst poisoning, suffocation, and Munchausen syndrome by proxy abuse are usually perpetrated by the mother. Abusing parents usually do not have an identified mental illness, though many show personality traits predisposing to violent behaviour or inappropriate sexual behaviour. Child abuse is more likely in those who are socially deprived and in families without a wage earner, but it is most important to recognise that it occurs in all layers of society.

Abuse is thought to be 20 times more likely if one of the parents was abused as a child. Though there is a strong tendency for those who were abused to abuse their own children in turn, more than a third of mothers abused as children nevertheless provide good care for their children and do not abuse them.

Awareness of the commonness of child abuse is an important step towards its recognition. The other necessary requirement is for doctors and nurses to be aware of the awful variety of ways in which children are abused. We can all understand the way in which a weary parent strikes an exasperating child but many normal people are too decent to imagine the degree of depravity, violence, cruelty, and cunning associated with child abuse. It is necessary to be aware of these wider limits because we can recognise and manage disorders only if we know about them from either experience or teaching. The chapters that follow will deal with both the common and the less common forms of child abuse.

Further reading

Department of Health. *Children and young people on child protecton registers year ending 31 March 1995, England.* London: Department of Health, 1995.
Feldman MD, Feldman MA, Goodman JT, *et al.* Is childhood sexual abuse really increasing in prevalence? An analysis of the evidence. *Pediatrics* 1991;88:29–33.
Finkelhor D, Dzruba-Leatherman J, Children as victims of violence: a national survey. *Pediatrics* 1994;94:413–20.
Kempe CH, Silverman FN, Steele BF, *et al.* The battered-child syndrome. *JAMA* 1962;181:17–24.
Department of Health. *The prevalence of child sexual abuse in Britain.* London: Department of Health, 1995.
Wisdom CS. Sampling biases and implications for child abuse research. *Am J Orthopsychiatry* 1988;58:260–70.

NON-ACCIDENTAL INJURY

Nigel Speight

> **Child abuse is the difference between a hand on the bottom and a fist in the face.**
>
> HENRY KEMPE

Difficulty of diagnosis

The diagnosis of physical abuse (non-accidental injury) is a difficult intellectual and emotional exercise. It is one of the most difficult subjects in clinical work, needing time, experience, and emotional energy. The biggest barrier to diagnosis is the existence of emotional blocks in the minds of professionals. These can be so powerful that they prevent the diagnosis even being considered in quite obvious cases (see, for example, case 1).

All those working with children should be warned that their overwhelming impulse on confronting their first case will be to want to cover it up.

The most important step in diagnosing non-accidental injury is to force yourself to think of it in the first place.

Importance of diagnosis

Non-accidental injury is one of the most important diagnoses in clinical paediatrics as it can so vitally influence a child's future life. At worst it is a matter of life and death for the child, and short of death there may still be possible brain damage or handicap. Though high risk cases are currently in a minority, the diagnosis remains crucially important in every case. This is because non-accidental injury is often a marker for emotional abuse and deprivation that can cause progressive and possibly permanent damage to a child's developing personality. This principle is especially relevant in children of school age. In such children the risk of death may be extremely small, yet non-accidental injury in older children is almost inevitably associated with a longstanding disturbance of the parent-child relationship. For this reason non-accidental injury should never be dismissed as "overchastisement".

Non-accidental injury is not a full diagnosis, it is merely a symptom of disordered parenting. The aim of intervention is to diagnose and cure (if possible) the disordered parenting. Simply to aim at preventing death is a lowly ambition.

In some cases the occurrence of physical abuse may provide an opportunity for intervention. If this opportunity is missed there may be no further opportunity for many years.

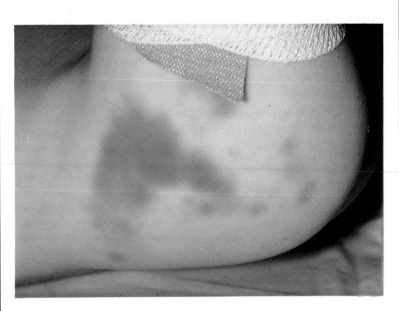

Case 1: The importance of what the child says

This 4 year old girl had been "rehabilitated" under a care order 8 months previously. She was brought to hospital with a fractured femur. Her father claimed that she had fallen down stairs, and despite the excessive bruising on her thigh and buttocks and her abject appearance no questions were asked. The next morning she told a nurse, "Daddy told Mummy he would never do it again". On further questioning the father became aggressive and had to be restrained by police from abducting the child after attempting to remove her Gallow's traction.

Diagnostic features

There are no hard and fast rules and no easy answers for diagnosis. The following list constitutes seven classic "pointers" to the diagnosis. None of them is diagnostic, neither does the absence of any of them exclude the diagnosis of non-accidental injury.

- There is a delay in seeking medical help (or medical help is not sought at all)
- The story of the "accident" is vague, is lacking in detail, and may vary with each telling and from person to person (innocent accidents tend to have vivid accounts that ring true)
- The account of the accident is not compatible with the injury observed
- The parents' affect is abnormal. Normal parents are full of creative anxiety for the

Case 2: The importance of the child's appearance

These pictures show the "before and after" effect when severe deprivation is reversed. This 3 year old boy was in fact never subjected to non-accidental injury, but many children in cases of non-accidental injury may have the same appearance. He was admitted after a genuine accident and noted to be extremely deprived. The bond between him and his mother was non-existent. (He had been admitted two years before with non-organic failure to thrive and retardation but allowed to lapse from medical follow up with no referral to social services.) In the ward he showed noticeable affection-seeking behaviour and flourished. The follow up photograph was taken six months later, while he was in foster care.

child. Abusing parents tend to be more preoccupied with their own problems—for example, how they can return home as soon as possible

• The parents' behaviour gives cause for concern—for example, they soon become hostile, they rebut accusations that have not been made, and they leave before the consultant arrives

• The child's appearance and his interaction with his parents are abnormal. He may look sad, withdrawn, or frightened (case 2). There may be visible evidence of failure to thrive. Full blown frozen watchfulness is a late stage and results from repetitive physical and emotional abuse over a period of time. The absence of frozen watchfulness does not exclude the diagnosis of non-accidental injury

• The child may say something (case 1). Always make a point of interviewing the child (if old enough) in a safe place in private. This is one of the virtues of admission to hospital. Interviewing the child as an outpatient may fail to let the child open up as he is expecting to be returned to the custody of the abusing parent in the near future.

Characteristic patterns of injury

Some forms of injury are by their nature virtually diagnostic of non-accidental injury.

These include finger tip bruising, especially when it is multiple (cases 3 and 4); cigarette burns and lash marks (case 5). In addition, torn frenula, unexplained subdural haematomata, and retinal haemorrhages (see pages 18 and 19) are highly suggestive of non-accidental injury.

How to approach a case of suspected non-accidental injury

Approach the parents as you would in any other clinical situation. Introduce yourself, shake hands, and proceed logically through the history, examination, provisional diagnosis, and decision making. Look at the "whole child", including other medical problems, and take a social history to form a picture of the family background. Look at the child's growth and development, since a degree of failure to thrive and impaired development due to neglect or emotional deprivation commonly coexist with physical abuse. Proper documentation at this stage will allow estimates of subsequent "catch up" growth and development to be made.

Try to avoid jumping to conclusions too soon. Proceed slowly and deliberately, keeping your mind open as long as possible. Avoid confrontation or accusing parents at this stage (although confrontation does have a part to

Case 3: Finger tip bruising and fractured ribs

This 4 month old baby was noted to have two bruises on the cheek highly suggestive of finger tip bruising from forceful gripping. A skeletal survey showed two healing rib fractures caused by an episode 4 to 8 weeks previously.

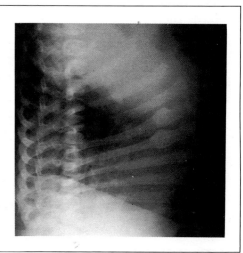

play in management once the diagnosis of abuse is definite).

Note keeping

The importance of good note keeping cannot be overemphasised, both for referring doctors and paediatricians. Discrepancies between first and subsequent accounts of the "accident" can be important when information is shared at a case conference, but need to be backed up by notes taken contemporaneously. Any medical notes may be scrutinised at a later date in a court of law, therefore loose or derogatory phraseology is best avoided.

Ideally all conversations with parents or caretakers should be recorded in full, and it is wise to have another member of staff present on each occasion as a precaution against subsequent complaints by the parents.

Bruises and other injuries should be described verbally and recorded diagrammatically with body charts. In addition, colour photographs should be taken whenever possible as they are such a vivid and accurate record of what has happened. Photographs can be very helpful in making the injuries real for case conference members, and

Retinal haemorrhage from non-accidental injury

are valuable as evidence in court. Subsequently they may enable a social worker to continue to confront parents with the reality of the abuse if they are attempting to minimise it.

Aging of bruises

Bruises of different ages are a common feature of abuse, and it is important to be able to give some estimate of the age of individual bruises without attempting to be too exact. The following is a rough guide for superficial bruises.

- <24 hours   red/purple
- 12–48 hours   purplish blue
- 48–72 hours   brown
- >72 hours   yellow

Bruises to avascular areas (for example, pinna of ear) or deep bruises may evolve at a slower rate than the above.

Investigations

When non-accidental bruising is suspected, blood tests should be performed to exclude medical causes for excessive bruising. These tests should include full blood count, clotting screen, and platelet function tests. Even when the case is obviously one of abuse the tests should be performed in case they are needed to support the diagnosis in future court proceedings.

Just occasionally, these tests will reveal a completely unexpected medical problem—for example, leukaemia or thrombocytopenia. Other medical causes of innocent bruising include cellulitis caused by *Haemophilus influenzae* or an apparent black eye from orbital deposits in neuroblastoma.

Skeletal survey should be performed in most infants and may reveal crucial evidence of previous bony injuries (see case 3). Repeat skeletal survey can be very useful in the follow up assessment of acute injuries as it may reveal previously unsuspected rib fractures and subperiosteal calcification of long bones in infants whose first skeletal survey was normal. It is much less appropriate in older children and should be used only in selected cases (page 10).

In all cases the local child protection register should be checked (usually via the duty social worker) to see if the child, or anyone else in the family, has been considered to be at risk or a source of concern to social services previously.

Case 4: Finger tip bruising

This 2 year old boy was admitted with a fractured tibia, bruising to the face, and classic finger tip bruising over the right scapula.

Case 5: Lash marks

This 10 year old girl was whipped with a belt by her depressed father. The linear nature of the marks is seen, together with a tramlining effect, in which the point of impact is white and the adjoining skin shows bruising caused by capillaries that have been broken by blood being forced into them.

Non-accidental injury

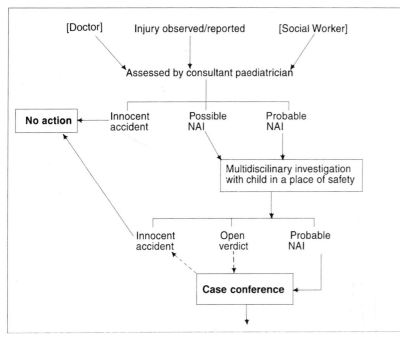

Flow chart for referral of cases of suspected non-accidental injury (NAI)

Hospital admission

It can be seen that hospital admission offers many advantages in the assessment, documentation, and investigation of suspected non-accidental injury. In obvious cases it allows a breathing space for social services in their decision making as the child is in a place of safety. In doubtful cases, it gives the paediatrician time to get the diagnosis right (see flow chart). It can also give valuable information from direct observation of parent-child interaction and parental visiting pattern.

Referral pathway

Most new cases of suspected abuse arise in the community and are brought to the attention of paediatricians by social workers. It should be emphasised that social services are the lead agency for the investigation and management of all forms of child abuse, with health professionals and police each having their part to play in what is essentially a multidisciplinary investigation. Local and national guidelines exist which doctors should familiarise themselves with and follow. The actual diagnosis of non-accidental injury, however, is predominantly the reponsibility of the doctor, usually the consultant paediatrician.

When the initial referral comes from a front line doctor the diagnosis of non-accidental injury is essentially a two tier exercise. The doctor on the front line (general practitioner, senior house officer in the accident and emergency department, or school doctor) is responsible for identifying children with suspected physical abuse and referring them to a consultant paediatrician for definitive diagnosis.

Role of front line doctors

Doctors on the front line must realise and accept the limits of their responsibility. They do not have to make a definitive diagnosis and should have a comparatively low threshold of referral. It should be accepted that some children with innocent injuries will be referred. If all of the children referred turn out to have been physically abused the threshold for referral is almost certainly too high.

Front line doctors should not feel guilt about referring children with suspected non-accidental injury to a paediatrician. They are not accusing either parent; they are simply asking for a second opinion on an important and difficult diagnosis. The fact that the child is being referred because of suspected non-accidental injury should be conveyed to the parents in a neutral and matter of fact way. It is not in the interests of children or parents for child abuse to be covered up. To do so leaves the parents at greater risk of inflicting more severe injuries next time, being imprisoned for causing more severe injuries, and losing long term custody of their children. Early intervention may help to prevent these events.

It is the duty of front line doctors to refer all children with suspected non-accidental injury. Failing to do so is a form of professional negligence. In the United States failing to report suspected child abuse is a federal offence punishable by imprisonment.

Role of the consultant paediatrician

It is vital to the interests of the child, the parents, and all the professionals concerned that the paediatrician reaches a correct and definite diagnosis in as many cases as possible. (This duty should not be delegated to junior staff.) If the paediatrician sits on the fence he or she will not only be in an uncomfortable position but also be doing a disservice to the child and the parents. If the paediatrician finds it impossible to decide initially he or she should admit the child to hospital while investigations continue. Few cases are uncertain after a thorough multidisciplinary investigation. The paediatrician should remember that he or she is being asked to commit himself or herself only on the balance of probabilities—not beyond all reasonable doubt. If the paediatrician genuinely cannot decide between non-accidental injury and an innocent injury, he or she should return an open verdict and decisions should be guided by the psychosocial assessment.

Further reading
Speight N. Bruises and burns: accidental or non-accidental. In: *Accidents and emergencies in childhood*. London: Royal College of Physicians, 1992:97–102.
Stephenson T. Bialas Y. Estimation of the age of bruising. *Arch Dis Child* 1996;**74**:53–5.
Schwartz AJ, Ricci LR. How accurately can bruises be aged in abused children. *Pediatrics* 1996;**97**:254–6.

FRACTURES

Chris Hobbs

Fractures are among the most serious injuries sustained after physical abuse. They may occur in almost any bone and may be single or multiple, clinically obvious, or occult and detectable only by radiography.

Prevalence

In one study of physically abused children more than half of the children (58%) were under 3 years old and they sustained most of the fractures (94%). In contrast, accidental fractures occur more commonly in children of school age.

The proportion of children presenting to hospital with fractures resulting from physical abuse rises to a maximum during the first year of life, when it may be as high as a half. A great deal of suspicion is required at this age. Most accidental fractures in infants and toddlers result from falls, although fractures are uncommon in falls of under 1 metre.

As early detection improves the proportion of children with fractures who are identified as having been physically abused falls from 50% to 10% or less. Most children with serious injury have suffered minor injury or shown other signs of abuse that have not been recognised or acted on by professionals in contact with the child.

Detecting fractures due to physical abuse

Children whose fractures are the result of an accident present crying excessively, with swelling or bruising, and are reluctant to use the affected part—for example, to put weight on a leg.

Some fractures caused by physical abuse are detected only by radiology because the fracture may be old, the physical signs having regressed; the site may be hidden—for example, the ribs, pelvis, or skull—and the parents will not have drawn attention to the possibility of injury.

Important patterns

Six important patterns are seen in fractures caused by physical abuse:
- A single fracture with multiple bruises
- Multiple fractures in different stages of healing, possibly with no bruises or soft tissue injuries
- Metaphyseal-epiphyseal injuries which are often multiple
- Rib fractures
- The formation of new periosteal bone.
- A skull fracture in association with intracranial injury.

As with all forms of physical abuse a careful history and examination and appraisal of the family potential for child abuse provides the framework for diagnosis.

Skeletal survey

The radiographic survey of the child's

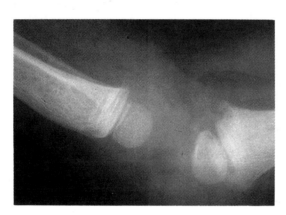

Metaphyseal (corner) fracture of lower end of femur in a child of 15 months who was swung by the legs and hit head against a wall

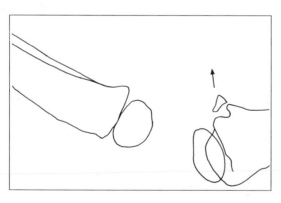

Distal metaphyseal chip fractures of lower end of tibia and fibula in abused infant

Fractures

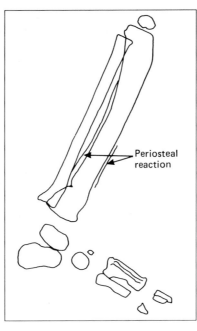

Periosteal reaction

Distal non-displaced fracture of lower shafts of tibia and fibula in abused child of 6 months, with evidence of periosteal reaction along tibial shafts. Fracture is probably 10–14 days old. Other injuries included multiple rib and complex skull fractures

skeleton must be complete. Babygrams (the whole baby in one radiograph) are generally unacceptable. Radionuclide bone scanning has a lower radiation dose and is generally more sensitive in detecting abnormalities (for example, rib fractures). It cannot detect healed injuries nor assess healing stages and may miss metaphyseal lesions around normally "hot" epiphyseal growth plates. Conventional radiography provides a high level of specificity and most injuries can be determined in this way.

Indications for skeletal survey

- Presentation with a fracture that suggests abuse
- Physically abused child under 3 years of age
- Older child with severe soft tissue injury
- Previous history of skeletal injury in child with suspected abuse
- Unexplained neurological symptoms or signs
- Child without an obvious cause of death (should be done early before necropsy and before bowel shadows obscure chest picture)

Specificity of radiological findings

No lesion is absolutely pathognomic of physical abuse but some carry higher specificity than others.

High specificity findings are metaphyseal or epiphyseal fractures, or both (corner and bucket handle fractures, chip fractures); rib fractures; multiple or wide complex skull fractures, or both; scapular and sternal fractures, which are uncommon; multiple fractures; fractures of different ages; and unpresented fractures.

Low specificity findings are single fractures; linear, narrow parietal skull fractures; fractures

in the shafts of long bones; and clavicular fractures.

Rib fractures

Rib fractures are usually occult and detected by radiography or radionuclide bone scanning. In infancy the ribs are very pliable and unless there is bone disease severe trauma can be implied.

Cardiopulmonary resuscitation is not responsible for fractures in this age group and unless an unusual history of direct thoracic trauma is given, abuse is extremely likely.

The fractures, frequently multiple, bilateral, and posterior, are thought to follow thoracic compression and distortion of the rib cage during shaking episodes or from kicks or blows in older children.

Metaphyseal and epiphyseal fractures

Metaphyseal and epiphyseal fractures are the classic injuries of physical abuse. Fragments of bone become separated from the ends of long bones either as a chip or as a whole plate. Such injuries arise from acceleration and deceleration as the infant is shaken by the body, arms, or legs. The forces of pulling and twisting applied to the weak metaphyseal areas of bone disrupt a fine layer of new trabecular bone close to the junction with cartilage. In epiphyseal lesions the injury occurs in the zone of hypertrophic cartilage with few radiological signs initially. The usual sites are the knee, wrist, elbow, and ankle. Metaphyseal lesions appear to cause little pain, tenderness, or swelling and heal without callus formation.

Fractures of the shafts of long bones

In assessing these injuries knowledge of the claimed and likely mechanism of production

Mid-shaft fracture of radius and ulna in 14 month old girl with old bruising to her thigh and failure to thrive. Fracture in itself carries little specificity for physical abuse, but bruising and growth chart (overleaf) greatly increase likelihood of physical abuse. Cohabiting boyfriend of girl's mother admitted swinging child by arm

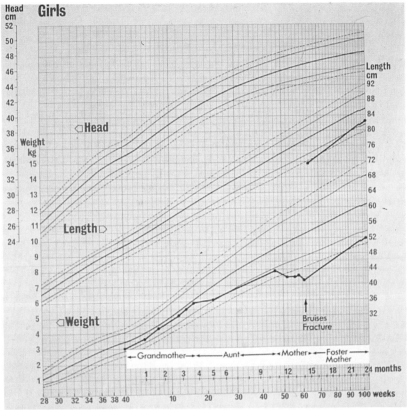

Growth chart of 14 month old girl with fractured tibia and fibula in case described on previous page. Pattern of failure to thrive developed from age of 4 months, when care was transferred to an aunt, and worsened when natural mother took over care at about 12 months. Catch up in length and weight were seen in foster mother's care. Children may react to changes in carer by developing behavioural difficulties, often centred on feeding, which may trigger violent responses from parents

may be useful: transverse fractures from angulation including from a direct blow; oblique transverse from angulation or bending with axial loading (compression); spiral from axial twists with or without axial loading; and oblique from angulation or axial twisting with axial loading.

Abuse injuries commonly arise when a limb is grasped, twisted, pulled, or used as a handle to swing or shake the child.

Certain fractures are commoner in

abuse—for example, humeral and femoral fractures in infancy, lateral clavicular, and small bones of hands and feet. Uncommon fractures with high specificity for abuse include fractures of the scapula, sternum, and spinal processes.

Spinal injury

Spinal injury in physical abuse usually results from hyperflexion-extension injury with damage to several consecutive levels. Defects in the lucency of the anterior superior edges of the vertebral bodies, often in the lower thoracic and upper lumbar regions, with narrowed disc spaces are characteristic. Multiple spinous process fractures are also described. Spinal cord injury may follow dislocation or subluxation.

Formation of new periosteal bone

Injury to an infant's developing long bone often results in subperiosteal haemorrhage, which raises the periosteum from the shaft while maintaining its firm attachment to the epiphysis. This process usually takes 10–14 days to appear and radiography may yield negative results initially. The finding may also point to an underlying fracture that is not easily visualised.

Such injuries probably arise when arms and legs are grabbed, pulled, or used as a handle for shaking the child. Trauma must be distinguished from other causes—namely, infection, Caffey's disease, vitamin A intoxication, leukaemia, and certain drugs—but all of these are far less common than physical abuse.

Dating fractures

Fracture dating is of obvious medicolegal importance. The table sets out peak times, although the earliest changes are sometimes seen a few days before this.

Resolution of soft tissue change	4–10 days
Periosteal new bone formation (earliest sign)	10–14 days
Loss of fracture line definition	14–21 days
Soft callus	14–21 days
Hard callus	21–42 days
Remodelling	1 year

From: Kleinman PK. *Diagnostic imaging of child abuse*. Baltimore: Williams and Wilkins, 1987.

The following should be noted:

• A fracture without periosteal new bone formation is usually less than 7–10 days old and seldom 20 days old
• A fracture with definite but slight periosteal new bone formation could be as recent as 4–7 days

Posterior healing rib fractures of left sixth, seventh, and eighth ribs behind cardiac shadow in abused infant. Presence of callus and unclear fracture line suggests fractures are at least two weeks old

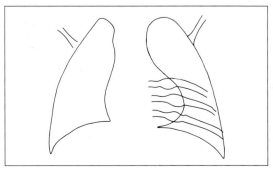

11

Fractures

Distal humerus epiphyseal separation in 5 month old infant with 25 separate non-accidental injuries, including five fractures. Initially injury was confused with dislocation but on follow up four weeks later extensive formation of medial new bone (right) confirmed displacement of epiphysis

New bone

Spinal injury in abused 6 year old child. Characteristic injury is present

 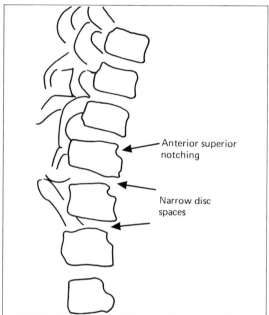

Anterior superior notching

Narrow disc spaces

● A 20 day old fracture will always have well defined periosteal reaction and typically soft callus

● A fracture with well developed periosteal new bone formation or callus is more than 14 days old.

Injury to the same (untreated) fracture may prolong healing and callus and fresh refracture may coexist.

Differential diagnosis of fractures

Child abuse is common. Non-traumatic causes of fracture or pseudofracture vary from uncommon to extremely rare. A balanced perspective is required if children's interests are to be preserved. Courts for the protection of children require probability rather than certainty in evidence.

Normal variants

The formation of new periosteal bone in infants and unusual suture lines in a skull radiograph could be normal variants.

Birth trauma

During breech deliveries the clavicle and humerus are often broken. If, however, callus is absent two weeks after birth the fracture did not occur during delivery.

Bone disease

Osteogenesis imperfecta—This inherited connective tissue disorder with abnormal collagen is occasionally confused with abuse as fractures are a major feature. There are a number of other features: bone fragility and osteoporosis; ligamentous laxity; skin fragility; blue sclera; dentinogenesis imperfecta; and presenile hearing loss.

In addition, a positive family history and wormian skull bones are features present in many cases. The condition is complex with four clinical types (I–IV), of which the rare IV is said occasionally to present clinically with little other than a fracture. This has been the basis of defence cases, although the incidence of this scenario has been estimated to lie between one in one million and one in three million births.

Copper deficiency—With osteogenesis imperfecta fractures should not suddenly cease when the child is removed to a safe environment, as they do in the case of abuse. Copper deficiency has been postulated as an explanation for temporary brittle bones in some cases of multiple fractures in infancy. Copper functions in various enzyme systems, deficiency resulting in sideroblastic anaemia, neutropenia, abnormal bones radiologically, hypotonia, and developmental retardation.

Bone abnormalities include osteoporosis, frayed and cup shaped metaphyses, and metaphyseal sickle shaped spurs, with changes distributed symmetrically throughout the skeleton. The condition occurs in low birth weight preterm infants, after prolonged total parenteral nutrition, after feeding milk deficient in copper (for example, doorstep milk), in malnutrition or malabsorption. The condition with fractures is rare. Skull and rib fractures have not been described. The plasma copper concentration is low.

Other conditions—These include prematurity (rickets), which may cause periosteal new bone formation and epiphyseal changes, which could be confused with abuse, or pathological fracture; scurvy; vitamin A intoxication; congenital syphilis; osteomyelitis; and neuropathic disorders.

Expert radiological, paediatric, and biochemical help may be required in occasional cases. The presence of a normal skeleton radiologically is strongly against the diagnosis of genetic, metabolic, or bone disease.

Further reading

Haller JO, Kleinman PK, Merten DF *et al*. Diagnostic imaging of child abuse. *Pediatrics* 1991;**87**:262–4.
Kleinman PK. *Diagnostic imaging of child abuse*. Baltimore: Williams and Wilkins, 1987.
Shaw JCL. Copper deficiency and non-accidental injury. *Arch Dis Child* 1988;**63**:448–55.
Silverman FN. Radiology and other imaging procedures. In: Helfer RE, Kempe RS, eds. *The battered child*. 4th ed. Chicago: University of Chicago Press, 1987:214
Spevak MR, Kleinman PK, Belonger PL, *et al*. Cardiopulmonary resuscitation and rib fractures in infants. A postmortem radiologic-pathologic study. *JAMA* 1994;**272**:617–8.
Taitz LS. Child abuse and osteogenesis imperfecta. *BMJ* 1987;**295**:1082–3.
Thomas SA, Rosenfield NS, Leventhal JM, *et al*. Long-bone fractures in young children: distinguishing accidental injuries from child abuse. *Pediatrics* 1991;**88**:471–6.
Warlock P, Stower M, Barbor P. Patterns of fractures in accidental and non-accidental injury in children: a comparative study. *BMJ* 1986;**293**:100–2.

HEAD INJURIES

Chris Hobbs

Head injury is the major cause of fatal outcome after physical abuse. The head is the commonest target for assault in the young child. In the first year of life 95% of serious intracranial injury is the result of abuse.

Two major categories of head injury described are: focal from impacts (punches, hitting the head from throwing or swinging the child on to or against an object or surface) and diffuse injury from acceleration-deceleration phenomena (shaking). A combination of the two is thought to account for many of the most serious injuries (the shaken-impact syndrome).

Between 40% and 70% of battered children have injury of some form to the face or head. These include bruises to the face or scalp;

traumatic alopecia and subgaleal haematoma; skull or facial fracture, or both; subdural and subarachnoid haemorrhage; cerebral contusion including diffuse axonal injury; intracerebral haemorrhage; and oedema. If the child survives, permanent physical and mental handicap may result.

Detecting head injuries due to physical abuse

When an infant rolls off a changing table, hospital trolley, cot, or bed, even on to a hard floor, serious injury rarely occurs. In one study 80% of infants escaped without any finding of injury whatsoever. The other 20% had a single cut, lump, or bruise. Skull fractures were found in 1%, and these were single and linear.

Extensive bilateral parietal fractures, which are wide and growing. Large lucent area represents surgical evacuation of large haematoma before 15 month old child died. Head was injured when the child was swung by the leg against a wall

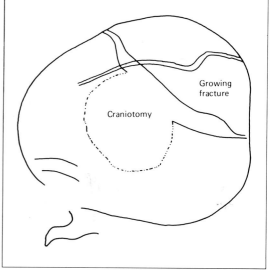

Growing fracture of parietal bone in 6 week old abused child. Father claimed to have dropped child, but old rib fractures and intracranial injury were inconsistent with history

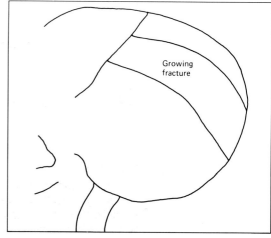

Manifestations of skull fractures

Child usually said to have fallen or banged head—for example, on door—or history may be absent

	Accident	Physical abuse
Type	Single linear	Multiple, complex, branched
Maximum fracture width	Hairline, narrow, 1–2 mm	Wide, growing, 3 mm or more
Site	Parietal One bone only	Occipital, highly specific Bilateral, parietal More than one bone affected
Depressed	Localised with clear history of fall on to sharp object	As part of complex fracture, extensive or multiple depressed areas
Associated intracranial injury	Unusual except after severe falls (2–3 m or more). Extradural haemorrhage uncommon but serious complication of simple fracture	Subdural haemorrhage, cerebral contusion, intracerebral haemorrhage, and cerebral oedema common

If an infant presents with a cranial swelling a day or two after a minor head injury and has a hairline parietal single linear fracture the cause is usually innocent provided that other injuries are not present

An equal number had a fracture at another site, of which the clavicle and humerus were the most common. No child sustained a subdural haematoma or life threatening condition. Falls from greater heights (between 1 and 2 m), as, for example, from a standing adult's shoulder, are more likely to result in a single linear parietal hairline fracture of the skull, and the infant may be irritable, vomit, or refuse a feed. Serious intracranial injury is extremely unlikely.

Even in more serious falls from heights in excess of 2 m or down stairs, when a fracture may show one or two features of abuse (table), serious intracranial injury is unusual. Occasionally, however, extradural haemorrhage can, if unrecognised and untreated, be fatal irrespective of the presence or absence of an underlying cerebral injury.

The force entailed in physical abuse—for example, in swinging the child, in violent uncontrolled shaking, and in hitting the child's head with a fist or foot or against a wall—is so much greater that the pattern of injury is different and serious intracranial injury results. Accidental intracranial injury in infancy is rare.

Scalp injury

The presence of injury to the scalp is often shown by a swelling, which can reach considerable size. This may represent bruising to the scalp tissues; if there is a fracture a subgaleal haematoma forms, into which much blood may be lost. Subgaleal haematoma also results from hair pulling as, for example, when a child is picked up by the hair. The swelling is diffuse and boggy and there are broken hairs with occasionally petechiae at the roots. There are no signs of scalp disease, such as loose hairs or scaling, which helps differentiate it from other forms of alopecia.

Skull fractures

Fractures indicate blunt impact injuries. Their reliable detection in a radiograph requires a radiologist or doctor experienced in differentiating usual and unusual suture lines in infants, which may be difficult. Swelling over the area helps, but the radiograph needs to be examined with bright light illumination.

The radiograph must be interpreted alongside the history. When there is a history of a minor fall, as is usually the case in infants and toddlers during the first two years, significant differences exist between the patterns of fracture after abuse and those after an accident. These are summarised in the table.

After abuse fractures tend to be extensive, multiple, complex or branched, depressed, wide, separated, and growing, and to cross individual suture lines, thereby affecting many individual skull bones. Whereas in accidents the parietal bone alone is usually affected by a single narrow linear fracture, in abuse other bones, notably the thick occipital bone and the base of the skull, are more likely to be fractured. Indeed, a fracture of the occipital bone should carry a high suspicion of abuse.

Growing fractures are not generally well known among doctors. These uncommon fractures occur only in infancy and entail a dural tear and brain injury beneath the fracture, which subsequently enlarges to form a cranial defect. Once a fracture reaches 0·5 cm in width in a radiograph it should be carefully followed for further growth. Such fractures seem to occur after a more severe blow to the head and are therefore more likely to be associated with abuse. Surgical treatment may be required to repair the defect.

Subdural haematoma

Subdural haematomas arise in over half of cases without the presence of a skull fracture. For a while they were termed "spontaneous subdural haematomas" until it was recognised that the infants had been abused. The evidence points to violent shaking disrupting bridging cerebral veins with bleeding into the subdural space, often over a wide area bilaterally.

In some cases the only additional evidence is the presence of retinal haemorrhages and there may be no bruising or other injury to the baby. These babies have been shaken violently, usually to stop them crying. Bouncing a baby up and down on a knee or an accidental head injury resulting in a simple

Subdural haematoma

fracture does not result in subdural haematomas.

Subdural haematomas arising after birth trauma produce signs and symptoms soon after delivery and should not lead to confusion. The concept of a chronic subdural haematoma after birth trauma is extremely dubious.

Children who develop irritability, vomiting, decreasing levels of consciousness, and irregular breathing or apnoea shortly after an alleged trivial head injury have probably been abused. Parents may admit to shaking the child mildly because "he didn't look too good" or "stopped breathing". In reality the child has been violently shaken. The diagnosis, once thought of, is most easily confirmed by computed tomography, but this can occasionally miss a difficult case.

Retinal haemorrhages

These are an important finding in non-accidental injury and are discussed in detail on pages 18–19.

Cerebral contusion, haemorrhage, and oedema

Cerebral contusion, haemorrhage, and oedema are responsible for many of the deaths and long term disability resulting from physical abuse. Areas of cerebral disruption, haemorrhage, and oedema are scattered throughout the brain, which swells, leading to a short term rise in intracranial pressure. Surgery is rarely helpful.

If the child survives, chronic disability is a real possibility. In one study Buchanan and Oliver estimated that between 3% and 11% of children residing in hospitals for those with learning difficulties were handicapped as a result of violent abuse. They described seizures and post-traumatic hydrocephalus, damage to visual pathways, and cerebral

infarction leading to atrophy and microcephaly.

Diagnosis of intracranial injury

When there is neither history of trauma nor obvious external signs of significant injury to the child, diagnosis may be difficult. A history of a minor household accident (for example, the child rolled off a settee or fell out of a baby bouncer) may be offered. The presentation may be with fits, unconsciousness, lethargy, and apnoea, and there may be delay in presenting the child for medical treatment.

Initially meningitis, encephalitis, infection, and toxic or metabolic disease may be considered the most likely diagnosis. Useful physical signs include a bulging fontanelle, low packed cell volume (indicating earlier injury), increasing head circumference, retinal haemorrhages, and torn frenulum.

Investigations

Lumbar puncture—May be bloody.

Skeletal survey (skull radiograph)—Look for fractures, widening of the cranial sutures.

Computed tomography—This is the examination of choice and is superior to magnetic resonance imaging in the acute stage for detecting subarachnoid haemorrhage and will also detect cerebral oedema and subdural haemorrhage. Both subarachnoid and subdural haemorrhage are thought to arise from disrupted bridging veins between the cortex and dural sinuses, with blood tracking into the interhemispheric fissure—this is well detected by computed tomography.

Magnetic resonance imaging—This is superior to computed tomography in detecting subdural haemorrhage as well as posterior fossa intraparenchymal injuries. Non-haemorrhagic white matter contusions and shearing injuries are also better shown, and dating of extracerebral fluid collections is enhanced. Also, the pictures are more impressive in court. It is important that T1 and T2 weighted sequences are used.

Cranial sonography—This is less sensitive than computed tomography.

Further reading

Billmire ME, Myers PA. Serious head injury in infants: accident or abuse? *Pediatrics* 1985;75:340–2.
Helfer RE, Slovis TL, Black M. Injuries resulting when small children fall out of bed. *Pediatrics* 1977;60:533–5.
Hobbs CJ. Skull fracture and the diagnosis of abuse. *Arch Dis Child* 1984;59:246–52.
Kleinman PK. Head trauma. In: *Diagnostic imaging in child abuse*. Baltimore: Williams and Wilkins, 1987. Chapter 8.
Levitt CJ, Smith WL, Alexander RC. Abuse head trauma. In: Reece RM, ed. *Child abuse. Medical diagnosis and management*. Philadelphia: Lea and Febiger, 1984.

OPHTHALMIC PRESENTATIONS

Alex Levin

Virtually any ocular injury may be the result of child abuse. Ocular injury is the presenting sign of physical child abuse in 4–6% of child abuse cases. Medical non-compliance and neglect can also result in permanent visual loss. Sexual abuse may be the route of transmission of a sexually transmitted disease to the eyes. Abused children may also develop functional symptoms such as blinking, unusual visual phenomena, or non-organic visual loss. Some people may consider the diagnosis of emotional abuse when parents or other adult caretakers allow children to view inappropriate materials, such as pornography or adult sexual behaviour.

Detection of ocular manifestations

Whenever a child less than 4 years old is suspected of being a victim of physical abuse, complete eye examination, including dilation of the pupil for retinal examination by an ophthalmologist, is essential. Examination with only a direct ophthalmoscope should not replace complete retinal examination, which can be accomplished only with the ophthalmologist's indirect (head mounted) ophthalmoscope. With indirect ophthalmoscopy retinal haemorrhages or other changes may be seen in the peripheral retina, which cannot be viewed with the direct ophthalmoscope. These findings, including peripheral retinal tears, may have particular importance in identifying the abused child. However, use of the direct ophthalmoscope by the primary care or emergency doctor can be a useful screening test. The pupils should be dilated with one drop of phenylephrine 2·5% and cyclopentolate 1% (except in premature infants, when cyclopentolate 0·5% is preferred). These drops may be repeated after 20 minutes if the pupils are not adequately fixed and dilated. If there is concern about using pupillary reactivity to monitor a child's neurological status, the cyclopentolate (duration of mydriasis up to one day) may be omitted. With phenylephrine alone pupillary reactivity should return in four to six hours. Despite the value of a positive direct ophthalmoscope examination, the absence of abnormalities, in particular retinal haemorrhages, does not obviate the need for consultation with an ophthalmologist. This is particularly true when shaking injuries are suspected. If an ophthalmologist is readily available it is best to forego pupillary dilatation unless he or she specifically requests it as he or she may wish to examine the child initially before pupillary dilation.

Child abuse must be in the differential diagnosis when any eye injury is evaluated. There are a number of ocular abnormalities which, when found, might suggest that trauma has occurred, even when a history to the contrary is given.

Whenever a child less than 4 years old dies suddenly for no apparent reason, gross and histological examination of the eyeballs should be included as part of the necropsy. Before removal of the eyeballs, an ophthalmologist, if available, may be asked to examine the child's retinas in situ to look for abnormalities such as retinal haemorrhages. Regardless of the result of the ophthalmologist's evaluation, both eyeballs should be removed, preferably along with the entire orbital contents from a

Ocular indicators of trauma		
	Result of injury	**Comment**
Eyelids	Laceration,* ecchymosis	Unilateral/bilateral ecchymosis may follow forehead trauma
Eyeball	Ruptured globe* (corneal/scleral laceration)	
Conjunctiva	Subconjunctival haemorrhage	Also from suffocation/strangle or abdominal or chest trauma
	Chemical burns	
Cornea	Scars	Especially bilateral acquired
Anterior chamber	Hyphema	
Lens	Cataract	Especially acquired unilateral
	Dislocated lens	Especially acquired unilateral
Vitreous	Haemorrhage Detached vitreous base*	
Retina	Haemorrhage, contusion* (Berlin's oedema, commotio retinae)	
	Retinal detachment	Especially if bilateral

* Pathognomic for trauma.

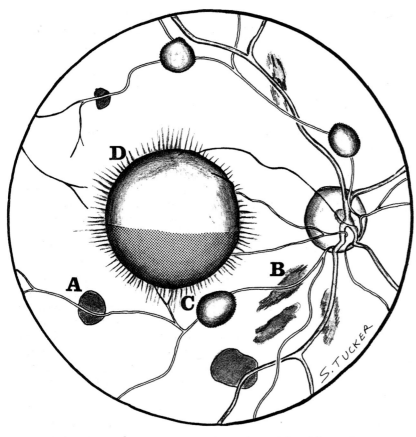

*An intraretinal blot haemorrhage—blood vessel passes into and through haemorrhage.
B Superficial flame shaped haemorrhage. C Preretinal haemorrhage—blood vessel obscured.
D Traumatic retinoschisis*

*Retinal haemorrhages in an abused child. Small arrows indicate superficial flame shaped
haemorrhages. Large arrows indicate "blot" intraretinal haemorrhages. No traumatic
retinoschisis is seen in this patient*

combined anterior and intracranial approach after removal of the brain. After fixation these tissues should be sectioned *en bloc*. Any gross or histological abnormalities should be photographed. If the pathologist is unable to remove the orbital tissues with the eyeball, then the entire globe, along with a long segment of optic nerve, should be removed from an anterior approach.

Consultation with an ophthalmologist may also be helpful in the following circumstances: conjunctivitis in a case of alleged child sexual abuse; suspected Munchausen syndrome by proxy with ocular signs or symptoms; the neglected child; and the abused child with visual complaints.

Retinal haemorrhages

Retinal haemorrhages are one of the cardinal signs of the shaken baby syndrome, occurring in about 80% of cases. These haemorrhages may occur in front of, within, or under the retina. They are usually bilateral. The exact mechanism by which they occur in the shaken infant is not clearly understood. Increased intracranial pressure; subdural or subarachnoid haemorrhage, or both; chest compression by the perpetrator's hand; and direct shaking injury to the retina or optic nerve may play a part. The intracranial approach to removal of the entire orbital contents, as described above, is designed to identify injury to the retina or optic nerve. Retinal haemorrhages in children less than 4 years of age are rarely caused by cardiopulmonary resuscitation with chest compressions or accidental head trauma. I am aware of only one convincing report of retinal haemorrhages secondary to resuscitation without other risk factors being present. These haemorrhages were few in number and confined to the posterior aspect of the retina around the optic nerve, unlike the retinal haemorrhages of the shaken baby, which tend to be distributed diffusely throughout the retina. Severe life threatening accidental head trauma (for example, that sustained in a road traffic accident), may, rarely, cause a small number of retinal haemorrhages in the posterior aspect of the retina. The type of accidental injury that would result in this clinical picture has an obvious history, eliminating any concern about child abuse.

Other systemic conditions can cause retinal haemorrhages in young children. They include acute hypertension, fulminant meningitis, vasculitis, sepsis, endocarditis, coagulopathy, leukaemia, and cyanotic congenital heart disease. Fortunately, these entities are usually easy to recognise from the history, a good physical examination, a complete blood count, and basic coagulation studies. Retinal haemorrhages are commonly seen after normal birth. Flame haemorrhages resolve in less than two weeks after birth. Large intraretinal dot/blot haemorrhages may, rarely, persist for up to six weeks. Diabetes mellitus and haemoglobinopathies such as sickle cell anaemia do not cause retinal haemorrhages in the age group most likely to suffer the shaken baby syndrome.

Traumatic retinoschisis is a form of retinal injury that may be virtually pathognomic of shaking injury. Owing to concomitant shaking of the vitreous gel which is adherent to the posterior retina in young infants the retinal layers are split apart to cause a dome shaped cavity, which may be partially or completely filled with blood. Some observers have described similar retinal abnormalities as subhyaloid haemorrhage—a collection of blood between the retina and vitreous gel. I believe this term may have been applied incorrectly in some cases as the clinical appearance of subhyaloid haemorrhage may be indistinguishable from superficial traumatic retinoschisis, an entity which has been confirmed histologically. Although this (posterior central retina), smaller cavities can be seen elsewhere in the retina, especially overlying blood vessels. When found over blood vessels these cavities do not seem to have as much diagnostic specificity. Although these lesions may heal with little visual result, circular folds and scars within the retina may serve as a marker of previous shaking injury. Other effects of shaking include retinal detachment and atrophy of the optic nerve.

Sexually transmitted diseases

The exact diagnostic significance of sexually transmitted diseases affecting the eye in non-neonatal prepubertal children remains somewhat unclear. Two retrospective studies have identified cases in which gonorrhoeal conjunctivitis was transmitted non-sexually. Gonorrhoea cannot be transmitted to genital or oropharyngeal locations by any route other than sexual contact. Perhaps the mucosal lining of the eye represents a special site in this regard. In all the cases of non-sexual transmission there was a family member who had a genital infection and a completely negative evaluation for sexual abuse (including negative cultures for other sexually transmitted diseases at other sites and an interview with the child by a person skilled and experienced in child sexual abuse).

Syphilis is the only organism that results in ocular effects exclusively through sexual contact. Although the presence of any other sexually transmitted disease should, at the very least, prompt consideration that possible covert sexual abuse has occurred, the possibility of non-sexual transmission to the eye of infections other than syphilis has not yet been disproved. With each of the infections, perhaps excepting ocular herpes and molloscum, a complete evaluation for sexual abuse is indicated. Reporting to child protection agencies should be reserved for those cases in which further evaluation confirms the suspicion of sexual abuse or fails to offer another plausible explanation.

Chronic and unusual visual symptoms or signs

Children may present with one of many functional ocular symptoms, including blinking, photophobia, eyelid pulling, eye rolling, and visual disturbances. Covert abuse is a rare cause of such symptoms but must always be considered when stress factors that are commonly associated with functional illness are investigated. Likewise, chronic ocular signs or symptoms such as recurrent conjunctivitis or abnormalities in pupillary size should provoke consideration of Munchausen syndrome by proxy in the appropriate clinical setting (page 47). In addition to these two signs, another case of Munchausen syndrome by proxy with ocular findings (recurrent periorbital cellulitis) has been described, and also nystagmus or strabismus from covert poisoning.

Further reading

Buys Y. Retinal findings after head trauma in infants and young children. *Opthalmology* 1992;99:1718–23.
Greenwald MJ. The shaken baby syndrome. *Seminars Ophthalmol* 1990;5:202–15.
Levin AV. Ocular manifestations of child abuse. *Ophthalmol Clin N Am* 1990;3:249–64.
Levin AV. Ophthalmologic manifestations of child abuse. In: Ludwig S, Kornberg A, eds. *Child abuse: a medical reference.* 2nd ed. New York: Churchill Livingstone, 1992.

Ocular manifestations of sexually transmitted diseases

Gonorrhoea*	Purulent conjunctivitis with possible spontaneous corneal perforation
Chlamydia†	Chronic conjunctivitis
Herpes simplex virus*	Keratitis, conjunctivitis, intraocular inflammation, retinal necrosis
Human papilloma virus†	Conjunctival papillomas
HIV*	Intraocular inflammation, retinal infections (for example, cytomegalovirus, toxoplasmosis), optic neuropathy, eye movement disorders
Syphilis	Intraocular inflammation, retinal vasculitis, optic neuropathy, eye movement disorders, and many other ocular abnormalities
Pubic lice†	Eyelash infestation
Molloscum*	Eyelid/periorbital lesions with possible secondary conjunctivitis

* Non-sexual transmission to eye in non-neonates documented.
† Route of transmission to eye not well studied.

BURNS AND SCALDS

Chris Hobbs

Accidental burns and scalds in children occur because of a lapse in the usual protection given to the child. Neglected children may be burnt because of inadequate or negligent parenting, which is a failure to protect the child, whereas in abused children burns and scalds are deliberately inflicted.

Burns and scalds within the range of child abuse are seen as serious injuries, as sadistic and linked with the sexual or violent arousal of an adult, and as punitive to evoke fear ("I'll teach him a lesson").

Prevalence

Deliberately inflicted burns and scalds are found in 10% of physically abused children, 5% of sexually abused children, and 1–16% of all children presenting at hospital with burns and scalds. This form of physical abuse is, however, underrecognised and underreported because diagnosis may be difficult.

The peak age of children accidentally burning or scalding themselves is during the second year; the peak age of children being deliberately burnt is during the third year.

Types of thermal injury

Scalds—These are caused by hot water—for example, in drinks, liquid food, and baths. Scalds cause blisters and the affected skin peels in sheets and is soggy and blanched. They have a characteristic shape: they follow the contours of clothes and are enhanced by them, and drip, pour, and splash patterns are seen. The depth of injury is variable and contoured.

Contact, dry burns—Such burns are caused by hot objects, usually metallic, and electric fires. The injury looks like a brand mark, sharply demarcated and with the shape of the object that caused it. The burn is dry and tends to be of a uniform depth.

Burns from flames—These are caused by fires and matches and may be identified by charring and by singed hairs.

Cigarette burns—These leave a circular mark and a tail if the cigarette was brushed against the skin. In physical abuse the burn tends to form a crater and to scar because the injury is deep. The injury may be multiple but is not particularly common.

Electrical burns—These are small but deep with exit and entry points.

Friction burns—These occur when, for example, a child is dragged across a floor. Bony prominences are affected and the blisters are broken.

Chemical burns—These may cause staining and scarring of the skin.

Radiant burns—These are caused by radiant energy—for example, from a fire or the sun. Injury is usually extensive and affects one aspect of an arm or leg or the body and is limited by clothing. The skin shows erythema and blistering. Such burns occur in children who are made to stand in front of a fire.

Left: Contact burns in 2 year old boy with developmental retardation who was abused by his mother. Burns to penis were also present.
Right: End of curtain wire heated in fire that was responsible for burns

Cratered deep cigarette burn in typical site on back of hand in 5 year old boy, who also said, "Mummy put her fingers in my bottom"

Depth of burns and scalds

The depth of burns depends on the temperature and duration of exposure. In the case of hot water immersion for adults the following serve as approximate guides:

- 52·7°C (127°F)—1 minute for full thickness scald
- 54·4°C (130°F)—30 seconds
- 65·5°C (150°F)—2 seconds

Above 60°C (140°F) children's skin burns in one quarter of the time of adult skin. The temperature of hot water in many homes as it leaves the tap is as high as 60°C (140°F), thus

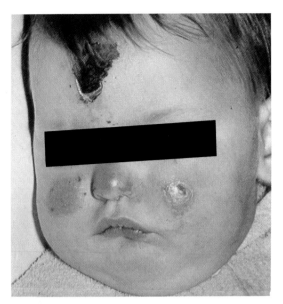

Friction burn in baby pulled across carpet by sibling

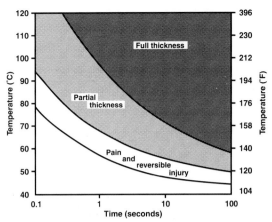

Relationship between temperature and duration of exposure and injury

Examination of this 18 month old girl's older brother in school for an unexplained burn on his back led to chance discovery of these old, healing, partially infected contact burns for which parents had not sought treatment. The source was fire; both children had been abused

SBRLSMD (Whitechapel)

increasing the risks of injury to children. In 1985 the Child Accident Prevention Trust suggested that the temperature should be set at 54°C. However, under the present BS 5546 specification for the installation of gas hot water supplies for domestic purposes, the maximum temperature of the cylinder thermostat and the BS 5549 maximum for forced circulation systems are both set at 60°C. In the United States new hot water heaters are set at 120°F (48·8°C).

Transfer of heat from hot water is more predictable than in other situations—for example, contact burns from hot objects. Obviously maintenance of close contact, with air excluded, will be prevented by rapid reflex withdrawal of the part, which cannot occur in

the same way with a scald. For this reason the mechanism by which contact was maintained must be ascertained in anything other than minor contact burns. Deep contact burns are likely to occur only when enforced contact has taken place.

Deep burns leave permanent scars which can provide later evidence of physical abuse.

History of physical abuse

In physical abuse the history of the burn is not consistent with the injury—for example, a 2 year old is said to have got into a bath of warm water, turned on the hot tap, and burnt both feet. There is a delay in seeking treatment or treatment is avoided altogether, the injury being discovered by chance.

The parent may deny that the injury is a burn when it clearly is and offer an unlikely explanation. The doctor may be told that the child did it to himself or that a sibling did. The incident is often unwitnessed ("I didn't see what happened, but he might have . . .") whereas in accidental injury to toddlers and young children parents are usually very clear what happened, even if they did not themselves see it.

A child who has been deliberately burnt may say that it did not hurt and the parent may tell the doctor that the child did not cry, which represents denial of what has happened. Alternatively, the child's history may disagree with that of the parents. The mother might

Left: Scalds from coffee thrown by drunken father at 3 year old girl producing scattered splash effect. Differentiation from accidental scalds from pouring liquids may be difficult

Right: Accidental scald typical of child pulling kettle from work surface by flex. Burn is variable thickness and head and shoulders take brunt of injury

Burns and scalds

Food burns in 9 month old child with failure to thrive that allegedly occurred when he was left alone with bowl of hot food. Parents' refusal to allow admission to hospital, absence of burns in mouth, and failure to match burn with supplied utensil left serious doubts

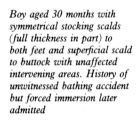

Admitted abuse in boy aged 3 years. Hand was held under hot tap

Extensive bath scalds in 3 year old girl failing to thrive. Central part of buttock spared where pressed on to cool base of bath—"hole in doughnut" effect. Abuse suspected but unproved

say that the child fell over on to the fire and the child tell a nurse quietly, "Mummy did it".

In physical abuse repeated burns are seen. In accidents once is usually enough for most parents and children.

Important sites and patterns
Accidental burns
Most common scalds in toddlers and older infants occur when the child pulls kettles, pans, or cups of hot water or drinks from a

kitchen unit or table. The scald affects the face, shoulders, upper arms, and upper trunk.

Accidental scalding from hot baths leaves an irregular mark with splashes.

Contact burns tend to be superficial, except in accidents with electric bar fires in which the hand sticks to the bar and sustains deep destructive burns to the palm.

Burns due to physical abuse
Non-accidental burns affect the face and head, perineum, buttocks and genitalia, the hands, and the feet and legs.

Cigarette burns may be seen on the face and head. Burns may be seen around rather than in the mouth when food has been pushed into the face.

To punish wetting and soiling misdemeanours or cure problems with wetting, abusing parents may dip the child's buttocks into a bath of hot water. The centre of the burn may show sparing where the buttocks pressed on the bath—the so-called "hole in the doughnut" effect. Burns to the perineum and genitalia may be part of sexual abuse.

Hands commonly show burns to the dorsal surface in physical abuse, whereas in accidents—for example, with an electric fire—the palm is affected. Hands are burnt by being held under a tap or on to hot objects.

The soles of the feet may show contact or cigarette burns. Burns on the feet and ankles may show a stocking or glove distribution with no splash marks and a clear tide mark when they have been caused by forced immersion in a sink or bath. Contact burns from fires (grid marks), irons, and curling tongs may also be seen on the legs and feet.

Characteristics of parents and children
Parents may be hostile, abusive to staff, and angry. They may refuse to allow the child to be admitted despite the need for treatment or threaten to discharge the child prematurely. Mothers who burn their children may be depressed, withdrawn, seeking help, and be themselves victims of child abuse (often sexual abuse).

In contrast with parents of accidentally burnt children abusing parents may show a

Boy aged 30 months with symmetrical stocking scalds (full thickness in part) to both feet and superficial scald to buttock with unaffected intervening areas. History of unwitnessed bathing accident but forced immersion later admitted lack of concern for the child or a lack of guilt. Parents of accidentally burnt children are often defensive, guilty, and dislike being questioned about the cause of the injury, which should not be misinterpreted as evidence of physical abuse.

A disturbed interaction between parent and child may show itself as anger and hostility towards the child—"It's his fault"—or as disregard of, or an inability to cope with, the child's behaviour. Abused children may be excessively withdrawn, passive, and uncomplaining about dressings or extremely anxious, hyperactive, angry, and rebellious, especially in the children's ward. In older children a reluctance to talk about their injury and how it occurred is worrying.

Assessment

Assessment is multidisciplinary and entails the participation of doctors (general practitioner, accident and emergency doctor, plastic surgeon, and consultant paediatrician), nurses, health visitors, social workers, police officers, and forensic scientists. In other words, the social services, the primary health care team, the hospital team, and the police need to liaise.

Visits to the child's home with the police may be required to inspect the bathroom, kitchen, fires, and household equipment.

History—This must be detailed and give the exact time of the incident, the sequence of events, and the action taken. Is the child's developmental ability consistent with what he

Inflicted contact burn on gas fire in 4 year old boy. Mother said dog knocked him on to fire when she was out of room. Child said that his mother did it. Burn was old and healing and was not presented for treatment. Child kept away from school

Partial thickness grid burn on back of wrist of 11 month old baby allegedly caused by older sibling. Mother later admitted responsibility for this single injury

is said to have done? For example, could an 18 month old child climb into a bath in the way stated?

Examination—Draw, measure, and photograph the injury. Manipulate the child's posture to discover his position when the injury occurred. Record the depth of the injury in relation to the temperature. Look for other injuries, and look for signs of sexual abuse during genital and anal examinations. Assess the child's demeanour, behaviour, and development. In physical abuse failure to thrive and a delay in acquiring language are common. Finally, always ask the child what happened.

Differential diagnosis

When there is a lesion and no history of a burn, skin infection or disease should be considered. Examples of conditions that may mimic burns are epidermolysis bullosa, impetigo, papular urticaria, contact dermatitis, and severe nappy rash.

Improbable accidents can occur. For example, a child could be burnt by vinegar as concentrated vinegar (glacial acetic acid) has a pH of 1·6. In addition, the buckles of seat belts or black vinyl seats heated by the sun have caused injuries that have been confused with physical abuse. In general central heating radiators are safe but hands have been badly burnt when they have been trapped behind one, and the injudicious use of hot water bottles for babies has resulted in burns that are caused by neglect rather than abuse.

Anaesthesia, an inability to move, or neurological deficit caused by a congenital insensitivity to pain, syringomyelia, spina bifida, mental disability, cerebral palsy, and epilepsy may be associated with unusual burns and scalds.

Neglect should also be considered. Children left alone at home have an increased risk of dying in house fires. Fireguards are required by law for children under 12. Negligent parents may fail to seek treatment when their children are burnt. Therefore the effects of neglect are serious and should also be reported to protective agencies.

Further reading

Feldman KW. Child abuse by burning. In: Helfer RE, Kempe RS, eds. *The battered child*. 4th ed. Chicago: Chicago University Press, 1987:197.
Hight DW, Bakalar HR, Lloyd J. Inflicted burns in children. Recognition and treatment. *JAMA* 1979;**242**:517–20.
Hobbs CJ. When are burns not accidental? *Arch Dis Child* 1986;**61**:357–61.
Lenoski EF, Hunter KA. Specific patterns of inflicted burn injuries. *J Trauma* 1977;**17**:842.
Yeoh C, Nixon JW, Dickerson W, *et al*. Patterns of scald injuries. *Arch Dis Child* 1994;**71**:156–8.

POISONING

Roy Meadow

A 3 year old child presented with recurrent seizures which did not respond to the usual anticonvulsants. She began to develop recurrent bouts of drowsiness. At first the mother denied giving drugs inappropriately but subsequently displayed them together with the container in which they were kept. When separated from her mother the child no longer had "seizures".

Accidental poisoning is very common; non-accidental poisoning is uncommon but more serious. Accidental poisoning usually occurs in toddlers aged 2 to 4 who explore the world with their mouth and try out any medicines, tablets, or other liquids that they find. The parent finds the 3 year old with an empty bottle in the bathroom or kitchen and is unsure how much the child has ingested. Usually the child has swallowed little or nothing and it is a poisoning scare rather than a true poisoning event. Less than 15% of the thousands of children presenting to hospital because of accidental poisoning develop symptoms from the drug; death is extremely rare. Death from non-accidental poisoning is more common.

Drugs that have been prescribed for the child, or another member of the family, are the commonest substances used to poison children. Anticonvulsants, opiates, and tranquilisers are particularly common. In contrast with accidental poisoning, intentional poisoning is often recurrent.

It is important to be aware that sometimes a parent, nearly always the mother, will have poisoned the child. Therefore the story should always be checked carefully for credibility—could such a young child have had access to those particular tablets? (Two year old children probably cannot reach the top shelf of the kitchen cupboard nor can they unwrap individually foil packed tablets or open child resistant containers. Child resistant containers are not childproof, but they do delay access to the contents, and when in doubt about the child's manipulative skills or development it is worth playing with the child to test their ability to open a container or pack of the type described by the parent.)

Detecting non-accidental poisoning

Intentional poisoning is commonest in children below the age of $2\frac{1}{2}$ but may occur at any age. Children who have been poisoned by a parent are likely to present in three main ways.

- The child presents with inexplicable symptoms and signs, usually of acute onset. These are summarised in the box on p 25, together with some of the drugs that have been given intentionally by parents to children.
- The child presents with recurrent unexplained illnesses that have the features in the box—for example, recurrent episodes of drowsiness or hyperventilation. These sorts of patients overlap with those for whom parents create false illness (Munchausen syndrome by proxy) by other means.
- The child may be moribund or dead when first seen by the doctor.

It is less common for the child to present in the usual way as a poisoning scare in which the parent rushes the child to hospital claiming that a drug or substance has been accidentally ingested. That presentation is more commonly associated with genuine accidents. In all cases, however, evidence of other forms of abuse or of sudden unexplained deaths in other children of the family should be sought.

Motive

A two year survey of non-accidental poisoning in the United Kingdom showed that two thirds of the cases occurred in the context of Munchausen syndrome by proxy abuse of

A notorious poison given by mothers is table salt—sodium chloride. An older child becomes thirsty, drinks plenty, and excretes excess salt speedily in the urine. But a younger child without access to water will be unable to do so. Then hypernatraemia develops leading to irritation, seizures, and coma. Death may occur. The high serum sodium concentration is associated with a high sodium concentration in the urine (unlike the urine of hypernatraemic gastroenteritis when the kidneys are retaining sodium and water). Hypernatraemia may lead to a confusing hyperglycaemia.

Symptoms	Drug
Seizures and apnoeic spells	Phenothiazines
	Tricyclic antidepressants
	Hydrocarbons
	Lignocaine
	Salt (sodium chloride)
Hyperventilation	Salicylates
	Acids
Drowsiness and stupor	Anticonvulsants
	Hypnotics
	Insulin
	Analgesics
	Tricyclic antidepressants
	Phenothiazines
	Methadone and cannabis
Hallucinations	Atropine-like agents
Bizarre motor movements (myoclonic jerks, tremors, extrapyramidal signs)	Phenothiazines
	Metoclopramide
	Antihistamines
Vomiting	Emetics and many other drugs
Diarrhoea (with or without failure to thrive)	Laxatives, including magnesium hydroxide (Milk of Magnesia) and phenolphthalein
	Salt
Haematemesis	Salicylates
	Iron
Ulcerated mouth	Corrosives
Thirst	Salt (with or without water deprivation)
	Lithium
Bizarre biochemical blood profile	Salt
	Insulin
	Salicylates
	Sodium bicarbonate

Characteristics of poisoning

	Accidental	Non-accidental
Age	2–4 years (rare $<1\frac{1}{2}$ or >5)	Any age
Presentation	Poisoning scare emergency	Unusual symptoms or illness
Substance	Usually a prescribed drug	Drugs; household or gardening product; berries or herbs
No of substances ingested	One	Sometimes more than one
Amount ingested	Usually none or little	Considerable
Symptoms	Uncommon	Common
Severe illness or death	Very rare	Less rare
Preceding unusual illness (factitious)	Absent	Common
No of episodes	One—recurrence rare	Recurrence common

the child by the mother. The other third occurred for various reasons, including parents seeking to "teach their child a lesson"; those who were themselves addicted to drugs, such as methadone or cannabis, and involved the child from an early age; and mothers who gave the child a drug to stop crying or enforce sleep.

Establishing poisoning

Identifying poisoning can be very difficult, even when the doctor is alert to the possibility. Most hospitals have a limited biochemical screen confined to major common drugs in urine samples; there is no fully comprehensive toxicology screen available. Therefore the doctor's job is, firstly, to think of possible drugs responsible for the child's symptoms; secondly, to try to identify from the general practitioner or hospital records any drugs that might be present in that household or to which the mother has access; and then, thirdly, to ask the laboratory to look specifically for that drug in the child's urine or blood. It is worth finding out if the parents' jobs give them access to particular drugs—for example, if one parent is a nurse or works in a hospital. Until such information is available samples of urine, blood, and vomit, if available, should be kept safely in the refrigerator. A few drugs are radio-opaque so a straight abdominal radiograph may be helpful if it is taken within a few hours of ingestion.

It is particularly important to preserve samples of urine, blood, and tissues when a child is brought in moribund with apparent encephalopathy, liver failure, bleeding disorder, or bizarre biochemical results. As urine is usually the most useful sample, it should be obtained if necessary by catheterisation or suprapubic aspiration. When such children die it is mandatory to inform the coroner. Whenever there is a strong suspicion of poisoning the police should be informed; their regional forensic laboratories can be helpful in analysing samples for they have more detailed screening systems, but even these regional laboratories cannot screen for everything, and they do their job best if they are given some idea of the type of drug to seek.

It is more important in the first place to try to identify the drug than the method by which the parent has given the drug to the child. Sometimes the methods are so bizarre that they defy the commonsense reasoning of a normal person. Parents do incredible things and a determined parent can find ways of poisoning a child, even when under the closest supervison. Mothers have injected insulin into intravenous lines, poured medicine into gastrostomy tubes, put nasogastric tubes down into the child's stomach to administer particularly noxious solutions that the child would otherwise not take, secreted tablets in their mouth that they have passed on to the child with a kiss, and secreted drugs behind the glass eyeball of the teddy bear they have

Poison information services

Belfast 01232 240503
Birmingham 0121 507 5588
Cardiff 01222 709901
Dublin 003531 8379964
Edinburgh 0131 536 2300
Leeds 0113 243 0715
London 0171 635 9191
Newcastle 0191 232 5131

There are six regional forensic laboratories in England and Wales, each serving six or more police forces, and the London Metropolitan Police has its own laboratory. In general their work comes directly from the police, though some will accept work from doctors through the local Home Office pathologist (whose name and address can be obtained from the local coroner's office)

given to the child. Rectal administration has been used also. The essential first step is to identify the poison and only then to start puzzling about how the child was given it.

If poisoning is suspected every chance should be given to the parent to explain how the child came to be given the poison. Many parents give drugs, tonics, and folk remedies to their child without telling doctors. Some are fearful of discussing it because they think the doctor would disapprove; others are embarrassed by trying a rather naive remedy for their child. Therefore the doctor should sympathetically explore with the parent the ways in which a child might have ingested a particular poison. This is particularly important for people from unconventional backgrounds or from different ethnic cultures, who may use many different sources of health advice.

Poison centres

Poison centres provide advice about drug overdoses, constituents of proprietary and household products, and also about treatment. They may also be helpful, when a child who has possibly been poisoned, by suggesting ways of identifying the drug.

Further reading

Dine MS, McGovern ME. Intentional poisoining of children. *Pediatrics* 1982;**70**:32–5.
McClure RJ, Davis PM, Meadow SR, *et al*. Epidemiology of Munchausen syndrome by proxy, non-accidental poisoning, and non-accidental suffocation. *Arch Dis Child* 1996;**75**:57–61.
Meadow R. Non-accidental salt poisoning. *Arch Dis Child* 1993;**68**:448–52.

FATAL ABUSE AND SMOTHERING

Roy Meadow

Despite the publicity given to violence and murder involving elderly women, police officers, or ethnic minorities, the person most at risk is the infant—by parental action.

Most forms of child abuse may at times lead to the death of the child. Head injuries are a particularly important cause of death as a result of a young child being shaken, hit, or hurled. Death also occurs, however, from severe burning, drowning, poisoning, and from starvation and neglect. Research suggests that the number of deaths from abuse has decreased in the last 20 years, mainly because of the work of child protection agencies.

Nearly all the fatalities occur in children below the age of 5 years and half of them in infants (age under 1 year). One reason is that infants are less robust and therefore more vulnerable to physical injury and certainly not able to either defend themselves against attack or fend for themselves if neglected.

Although many parents worry about their child being attacked or murdered by a stranger, and such events achieve massive publicity, they are rare. When a child is killed the usual perpetrator is the child's parent or carer. *Filicide* is a term used to describe the killing of a child by a parent or step-parent.

Similarly the well publicised family annihilator who kills himself, his partner, and his children is a rare phenomenon. On the other hand, child abuse is one of the common causes of death in infants and characteristically is perpetrated by a parent in the home; collusion between two parents is rare, and it is more common in stressed families with low socioeconomic status, in young mothers, and after unwanted pregnancies.

The reasons for the killing range from those in which there is no intention to kill or harm to those in which the parent views the child with anger or jealousy, the parent who has ill-founded ideas of discipline, and parents with

frank psychosis. Fatal poisoning and smothering are much more likely to be perpetrated by the mother than the father. Although British law defines infanticide as the killing of a child under the age of 12 months by the child's mother "when the balance of her mind was disturbed because she had not fully recovered from the effect of child birth or lactation", most mothers who kill are not found to have mental illness when subject to expert assessment by psychiatrists. Most, however, do have personality disorders and are reacting to difficult circumstances, including poverty, lack of supporting family and friends, and the demands of awkward children. If the parent herself comes from a background of family violence and one where there is drug or alcohol dependence the risks are even greater.

Such deaths can be seen as the extreme end of most forms of child abuse and, in that way, may be understood. But a much more difficult subject is the covert killing in which a young child dies suddenly and there is uncertainty about the cause. In recent years there has been greater recognition of this occurrence and a willingness to confront the issues. The difficulty has been to do this in a way that is sensitive to the feelings of the parents who suffer the tragedy of a young child dying, suddenly and unexpectedly, from natural causes.

The sudden infant death syndrome—cot death

The label is used when a previously well infant dies suddenly and unexpectedly, neither the preceding history nor the necropsy suggesting a cause of death. The campaigns to improve safe conditions for young children, including putting the infant to sleep supine, appropriate bedding, and avoiding overheating and smoking, as well as advances in the early detection of illness, have contributed to a decline in the numbers of babies dying suddenly. It is still, however, the commonest category of death in Britain for infants aged between 1 month and 1 year, particularly in the 2–5 month age group, and the usual circumstance is that the infant is put down to sleep at night and then found dead the next morning. Various reasons probably account for these deaths. There do not seem to be specific genetic factors entailed and so there is no reason to expect recurrence within a family.

It has long been recognised that a small proportion of such deaths are the result of the

Fatal abuse and smothering

A healthy baby was born by normal delivery at full term. At the age of five weeks he was rushed to hospital after a 999 call because of stopping breathing. Examination and investigations were normal. Three days later he was discharged home but returned to hospital that evening having had a further bout of apnoea. Although he was in a collapsed condition, he recovered speedily and appeared normal during the next seven days in hospital. A barium swallow examination revealed some gastro-oesophageal reflux, but he did not vomit or regurgitate feeds while in hospital. Other investigations were normal. He was discharged home with an apnoea alarm but died the following weekend, his mother having fed him at 1.00 pm and then, one hour later, hearing the alarm and finding him dead on the sofa. Necropsy revealed no cause, the coroner was informed, and the death certified as the sudden infant death syndrome.

Almost exactly two years later the mother's second child began to have similar episodes of apnoea. During the course of investigation in hospital the baby was observed kicking and struggling violently as his mother pressed a pillow on his face.

parent's actions (acts of commission as well as omission). And as many of the natural causes of the syndrome have been eliminated and mortality has fallen it has meant that the proportion caused by parents has gradually increased. Some deaths are caused by deliberate acts such as suffocation, others result from poor care and neglect which may or may not be deliberate. The work of the National Advisory Body for the Confidential Enquiry into Deaths in Infancy suggests that between 10% and 20% of all sudden unexpected deaths in infancy are likely to arise from parental action.

Smothering

Asphyxia is an uncommon but serious form of child abuse. At best, if brief it may merely be a terrifying ordeal for the child. If the period of brain hypoxia is prolonged, however, permanent brain damage or death may result. The commonest method is by smothering; the abuser, usually the child's mother, using her hand, a pillow, or a pad of clothing to cause mechanical obstruction of the child's airways. Less commonly she presses the child's face against her chest, uses a plastic bag, or strangles by pressure on the child's neck.

Clinical features

Smothering is commonest under the age of 1 year and rare over the age of 3 years. The infant presents to doctors either as a sudden unexplained death, moribund (near miss cot death), or as a single or recurrent episode of being found cyanotic, floppy, and having stopped breathing. The mother's account leads doctors to diagnose an apnoeic attack or a seizure. (If a mother describes a young baby as having stopped breathing or having seemed unconscious for a short time the doctor usually calls it an apnoeic attack whereas in an older child the same description is likely to gain the label of a seizure.) For some children the smothering is associated with other forms of child abuse, particularly physical abuse and Munchausen syndrome by proxy. The British survey into the incidence of suffocation identified mainly the severe and repetitive

cases and found that half of those occurred in the context of Munchausen syndrome by proxy abuse, the child being presented to doctors repeatedly because of apnoea or collapses. When such an infant is being presented repetitively because of "stopping breathing" there is usually a mixture of events, some of which are merely false stories, and other events which the mother has caused by smothering after which the child may have been found, by experienced observers, to be blue or lifeless. Single acts of smothering, even if fatal, are unlikely to be detected.

Warning features that a sudden infant death may have been caused by a mother smothering her child are:

- Previous episodes of unexplained apnoea, seizures, or "near miss cot death"
- An infant aged over 6 months
- Previous unexplained disorders affecting that child
- Previous unexplained disorders affecting siblings
- Other unexplained deaths of children in the family
- Death on the anniversary of a previous child's death.

Secondary features that add to the concern are:

- A mother who predicted the death of the child or the event
- An excess of unusual illnesses during the mother's pregnancy
- A child who suffers a severe episode, or dies, within 36 hours after being discharged from hospital
- A child who at necropsy is found to have coins, paper, or other foreign bodies in the stomach or intestine
- Parents who have an unusual response to the child's life threatening episode or death, including bizarre mourning rituals.

Signs of smothering

Smothering is violent: a young child who cannot breathe struggles and tries to get air. Characteristically the mother lays the child on his back, or against something firm, so that the hand or cushion may be held hard against his face. The smothering probably has to persist for at least a minute to cause seizures, longer to cause brain damage, and over two minutes to cause death. (Damage may be more sudden if the child, as a result of the assault, has a cardiac arrest or vomits and chokes). Despite the violence entailed, signs may be non-existent or few. Hand pressure sometimes leaves thumb marks or finger prints around the nose or mouth or abrasions inside the mouth with bruising of the gums. Sometimes the asphyxiation leads to multiple petechiae on the face, particularly on the eyelids, as a result of the raised blood pressure, lack of oxygen, and retention of carbon dioxide. All forms of asphyxiation may be associated with some bleeding from the nose or mouth, but it is not inevitable. Immediately after a bout of severe

And Then There Were None

During their 14 years as parents, Mary Beth and Joseph Tinning buried nine children. Until the last death, authorities never suspected wrongdoing. How could this happen?

THE GUARDIAN
Friday December 2 1988

First child 'smothered,' said mother

Upstate Mother Is Held

A MOTHER accused of murdering her second child, who was dropped, kicked... her first...

smothering the baby when met her with a young man ... hostel... Miss Mo...

Continued From Page 1 –

2-year-old had been hospitalized for what was called a fall down a flight of stairs. Social service...

After 9 Babies Die in 14 Years, Mother Is Held

By AMY WALLACE
Special to The New York Times

...ADY, N.Y., Feb...
...me after...

It was not until Wednesday, when the ...ice charged Mrs. Tinning, who is 43 ...old, with ...focating her ...ted dau...

said there might have been incomplete examinations of the deaths and lapses ...communication among docto...

hypoxia the infant commonly has an increased respiratory rate, sometimes pulmonary oedema on a chest radiograph, and non-specific signs of extreme stress such as hyperglycaemia and raised blood white cell count. Usually recovery to normal is rapid.

Fatal smothering may be associated with no external signs, and at necropsy there may be no specific signs that enable the most experienced pathologist to differentiate the death from the sudden infant death syndrome. Some of the children who have suffered recurrent bouts of smothering have evidence of previous bleeding into the lungs and an excess of haemosiderin deposits. Some may have more specific evidence of brain damage from anoxia, but most will not have specific pathological evidence of smothering. Thus, there has to be careful exploration of all the circumstances and previous history when the cause of death, is considered.

Differential diagnosis

Unexplained episodes of apnoea or a seizure are commonly reported by mothers of young babies. Sometimes an anxious mother perceives illness that is not there or overinterprets the periodic breathing and normal movements of a healthy baby. Therefore in all such cases it is worth seeking a description of the episodes from another relative. This is particularly important if the mother is suspected of causing the episodes.

True apnoea, in which the breathing stops for 20 seconds or more and is followed by bradycardia, cyanosis, or pallor, is frightening and often unexplained. It is more likely in small preterm infants and usually starts in the neonatal period. In early life both respiratory syncytial virus infection and whooping cough can be associated with spells of apnoea in previously well infants; the apnoea may precede the cough or other respiratory signs by a few days.

Whenever apnoea starts unexpectedly in a previously well baby it must be investigated thoroughly. The investigations should include careful checks for cardiac or respiratory disorder, oesophageal reflux, and a biochemical or seizure disorder. When these investigations give normal results consideration should be given to whether the episodes are being caused by the mother; if the episodes are frequent a period in hospital without the mother might be the wisest course. If the episodes are frequent at home and absent in hospital away from the mother, the mother is probably responsible. Some hospital units are able to arrange covert video recording of the infant and mother in hospital. As a diagnostic test video surveillance is highly specific as filmed evidence of suffocation provides conclusive proof. But it is not very sensitive as most abuse occurs at home and even if the mother does suffocate her child in hospital she may well not do so during the period of video surveillance.

Those providing a highly specialised service for children with alleged recurrent apnoea and sleep apnoea and who issue apnoea alarms and monitoring equipment to such families are particularly likely to encounter children incurring repetitive smothering.

There is now substantial experience of mothers who repetitively smother consecutive children, and reports of mothers killing 3—or even 9—children. "One sudden infant death is a tragedy, two is suspicious and three is murder until proved otherwise" is a crude aphorism but a sensible working rule for anyone encountering these tragedies.

Further reading

Special issue on fatal child abuse. *Child Abuse Review* 1995;**4**:309–392.

Working party of the British Paediatric Association. *Evaluation of suspected imposed upper airway obstruction.* London: British Paediatric Association, 1994.

Meadow R. Suffocation, recurrent apnea and sudden infant death. *J Pediatr* 1990;**117**:351–7.

Samuels MP, McClaughlin W, Jacobson RR, *et al.* Fourteen cases of imposed upper airway obstruction. *Arch Dis Child* 1992;**67**:162–70.

Department of Health. *Third annual report of the confidential inquiry into stillbirths and deaths in infancy (CESDI).* London: Department of Health, 1996.

EMOTIONAL ABUSE AND NEGLECT

David Skuse

Emotional abuse and neglect of children may take many forms, from a lack of care for their physical needs, through a failure to provide consistent love and nurture, to overt hostility and rejection. Deleterious effects on developing children are correspondingly diverse and tend to vary with age. In infancy neglect of physical care is likely to produce the most obvious consequences and developmental delays are also found. Preschool children may additionally present with disorders of social and emotional adjustment. Older children are likely to show behavioural problems at school, which are often accompanied by extensive learning difficulties. Emotional abuse is rarely the sole reason for seeking child protection through legal action, yet evidence is accumulating that its long term consequences on social, emotional, and cognitive development may be far reaching and profound. There is growing awareness that not only do many, if not most, cases of physical abuse and neglect occur in a context of emotional maltreatment, but it is the psychological aspects of the maltreatment that are of the greatest significance for future adjustment.

Neglect comprises both a lack of physical caretaking and supervision as well as failure to engage the developmental needs of the child in terms of cognitive stimulation. Although direct observation of parenting may raise suspicions about the presence of emotional abuse and neglect, the diagnosis is usually suggested by its consequences in the child: "the severe adverse effect on the behaviour and emotional development of a child caused by persistent or severe emotional ill-treatment or rejection".[1] All abuse entails some emotional ill treatment. There is often accompanying physical or sexual abuse. Without signs of physical or sexual maltreatment and disclosure of specific abusive activities, however, it is still possible to recognise characteristic groups of features that demand further investigation. Current knowledge on the subject does not yet allow us causally to link specific patterns of maltreatment to particular delays and disorders. In addition, the symptoms and signs to be described are not invariably indicative of abuse and neglect. But the cessation of abuse and its substitution with sensitive care—often in an alternative home— is usually followed by a rapid and dramatic improvement in developmental attainments, behaviour, and socioemotional adjustment.

Defining features

Emotional abuse refers to the habitual verbal harassment of a child by disparagement, criticism, threat and ridicule, and the inversion of love; by verbal and non-verbal means rejection and withdrawal are substituted.

Infants

Neglect of the physical and emotional nurture of an infant is likely to result in various signs and symptoms that should be fairly easily recognised. The aspects of physical development that are affected are those that demand the closest attention from caregivers. Babies are dependent creatures: they need to be fed regularly, to be kept in a reasonably dry and warm environment, and to have their bowel and bladder functions taken care of. If they are habitually cold and wet they will contract recurrent infections; if they do not have their nappies changed regularly they will develop nappy rash, which if neglected may cause scarring; if they are not fed adequately they will fail to thrive. Failure to thrive is usually defined as an exceptionally poor rate of growth in which weight (and often length) becomes increasingly divergent from normal age standardised values in the population. There are many reasons why such a pattern of growth may occur. Recent population surveys show that it is only exceptionally associated with abuse or deliberate neglect—even in non-

---

Key features in infants

Physical	Failure to thrive
	Recurrent and persistent minor infections
	Frequent attendances at casualty departments or admissions to hospital
	Unexplained bruising
	Severe nappy rash
Development	General delay
Behaviour	Attachment disorders: anxious, avoidant
	Lack of social responsiveness

organic cases. In families in which abuse is suspected other evidence to support those suspicions should be sought.

When there has been serious neglect social and psychomotor skills are also likely to be affected. If there has been no encouragement to acquire skills such as sitting, crawling, and walking the infant may show developmental delay. Infants are innately sociable: they enjoy interacting with others, adults or children. A severely neglected infant will not have learnt the joy of reciprocal smiling and laughter and so may not try to elicit attention. Although the concept of infant depression is controversial, increasing evidence suggests that the infants of some depressed (and therefore comparatively neglectful) mothers do show characteristic social responses, such as withdrawal, "looking away" behaviour, and emotional flattening. There may be long term adverse consequences for the child's cognitive development too, boys being especially vulnerable. Severely understimulated infants may use self stimulatory behaviours such as persistently banging their head or rocking.

Selective attachments to important adults in an infant's life begin to be established around 6 to 8 months of age. A neglected or abused infant may show an unusual pattern of attachment. Usually the experience of consistent and sensitive parenting leads a child to feel safe and secure with the primary caregiver, even in the presence of a stranger. In an unfamiliar setting such as a surgery or clinic the wish to explore will be counterbalanced by a wish to stay close to the parent. Infants who have been abused or neglected lack this sense of security. They do not have sufficient confidence to explore their surroundings and seem ill at ease, whining and unhappy, and cling to their caregiver, who responds with irritation. Alternatively, there may be little evidence for any attachment behaviour and the infant either roams around the room in a completely non-directed fashion (attributable perhaps to high anxiety) or creeps quietly into a corner and observes the proceedings warily (frozen watchfulness). Recent research has shown, however, that large differences in the availability of, and

nurture by, a caregiver do not always correlate with variations in attachment.

Preschool children

The physical consequences of persistent abuse and neglect through the preschool period often include poor growth, not only in height and weight but also in the circumference of the head. Dramatic increases in head size have been documented when abused children have been removed to a nurturing alternative environment. Associated indicators of abuse include recurrent minor unexplained injuries, especially bruising. It is important to be aware of the distribution of bruises that is likely to indicate squeezing, choking, and slapping.

The development of communication between children, even those who cannot talk, and their caregivers is a subtle process with its own set of shared expectations and rules of operation. Persistent neglect and abuse will prevent the establishment of a "mutual faith in a shared world". Retardation in the development of receptive and expressive language will result, possibly exacerbated by recurrent inadequately treated middle ear infections and partial deafness. When the emotional abuse has been severe a child may become virtually mute. Language development seems to be especially vulnerable to the effects of a severely depriving environment.

The main indicators of emotional abuse and neglect of preschool children are usually behavioural. As long as the child does not mix in a social setting no problems may be reported. In a nursery school or day nursery, however, the child may show many and characteristic disorders. Attention span is commonly extremely limited: the child cannot settle to any task for more than a few seconds. This probably reflects a lack of attempts to engage the child's attention at home, but it may also indicate profound anxiety. Poor attention is often associated with excessive activity: such children may be described as hyperactive, although there is no evidence that most overactive preschool children have been abused. Aggressive disorders of conduct are an additional problem, and children who are observed persistently to hit or swear at their caregivers in the consulting room must be regarded as being at risk.

Peer relationships will inevitably be problematic as persistently abused children do not develop sufficient social maturity to play cooperatively. Therefore their relationships with other children may be characterised by a combination of aggression and withdrawal. Social relations will also be impaired by a lack of selective attachments; thus abused toddlers may show indiscriminately friendly behaviour that is qualitatively different from that seen in children who are merely temperamentally predisposed to be sociable. It is also unlike the open, friendly behaviour shown by children with broad social experience. In contrast, such children elicit intimate physical contact from

compl strangers.

Key features in preschool children

Physical	Short stature
	Microcephaly
	Unkempt and dirty
Development	Language delayed
	Attention span limited
	Socioemotional immaturity
Behaviour	Overactive
	Aggressive and impulsive
	Indiscriminate friendliness
	Seeks physical contact from strangers

complete strangers—they may end up on your lap within a few minutes of meeting—and seem to crave physical contact ("touch hunger"), even in the presence of their primary caregiver.

School children

In the child who has reached school age the effects of long term abuse and neglect occasionally lead to a diminution in their rate of growth in height, which is often associated with disorders of appetite and sleep. In many cases, however, there is no evidence of an effect on growth and the main indicators of abuse are to be found in poor social and emotional adjustment, behaviour problems, and learning difficulties.

School may be unable to compensate for the long term lack of cognitive stimulation at home because abused children have tremendous problems attending to learning tasks. The failure in concentration is often coupled with physical overactivity of such a degree that the child is regarded as disruptive and may be referred for assessment for special education.

Persistent denigration and rejection will inevitably cause a lowering of self esteem; children who feel they are worthless often carry a huge burden of guilt for their "bad" behaviour. They may seem depressed and persistently apologise for trivial and meaningless supposed misdemeanours. For example, an abused 5 year old seen recently at her first visit to a child guidance clinic apologised to the therapist for not having saved him a piece of her birthday cake; her birthday had been three months previously. Such a poor self image is not really compatible with forming and keeping friendships at school; the social skills needed to negotiate such relationships have never been learnt. Thus the emotionally abused child stands alone at playtime or is seen drifting around the periphery of small groups engaged in their own pursuits. Sometimes more able children develop a coping strategy whereby their main social interaction is with adults—that is, with teachers rather than pupils. They show a pseudomaturity that belies their lack of sense of self worth and their longing for affection and stability. When the abuse has been coupled with a style of interaction that is aggressive and threatening the child may show similar behaviour, directed towards pupils and teachers. Such behaviour may also be habitual because at home it is the only way of attracting attention.

In extreme cases of emotional abuse and neglect patterns of behaviour are so unusual or bizarre that they inevitably draw attention to the child. Self mutilation, from skin picking to deliberate self injury with knives or glass, is one. Others include repetitive rocking or other self stimulatory activities, including sexual behaviours. Unusual patterns of defecation or urination are worrying in school children. Children who urinate or defecate in their clothes in class may be shunned as being smelly by their peers; perhaps that is how they view themselves—as disgusting and unpleasant individuals. Pools of urine or piles of faeces in the corridor or playground are signs that the culprit is urgently in need of assessment for possible abuse.

Adolescence

Adolescent abuse is less well recognised than it should be; recent research suggests that up to half of all abusive incidents involve this age group but they are far less likely to be reported to protection services than their equivalent among younger children. All forms of maltreatment do occur, but sexual and psychological abuse predominate. Girls are more likely to be victims as they pass through adolescence than during earlier childhood, whereas boys are at greater risk at a younger age. A substantial number of abusive incidents have their onset at this time; they are not simply the continuation of an earlier established pattern of behaviour. In contrast with the picture of abuse and neglect in early childhood all socioeconomic groups are equally at risk, but families with step-parents are especially vulnerable. The detrimental consequences of psychological, sexual, and physical maltreatment on adolescent adjustment may be severe. An association has been found with contemporaneous and later suicide attempts, drug and alcohol misuse, running away, promiscuity, and delinquency.

Investigation and management

Children who are being emotionally abused or neglected may not be in immediate physical or moral danger, but their need for protection is not, for all that, diminished. It must be acknowledged, however, that there is limited scope in such cases for medical investigation in the absence of associated physical or sexual maltreatment. Doctors who suspect that a child is being emotionally abused should first seek the advice of a colleague who is

---

Key features in school children	
Physical	Short stature
	Poor hygiene
	Unkempt appearance
Development	Learning difficulties
	Lack of self esteem
	Poor coping skills
	Socioemotional immaturity
Behaviour	Disordered or few relationships
	Self stimulating or self injurious behaviour, or both
	Unusual patterns of defecation or urination, or both

experienced in such matters. If no local paediatrician or child psychiatrist is available an inquiry to a tertiary referral centre elsewhere in the country will often be met with a courteous and helpful response. Subsequently, it will be necessary to share concerns with the statutory services responsible for child protection.

1 Department of Health and Social Security and the Welsh Office. *Working together under the Children Act 1989. A guide to arrangements for inter-agency cooperation for the protection of children from abuse.* London: HMSO, 1991.

Further reading

Downey G, Coyne, JC. Children of depressed parents: an integrative review. *Psychol Bull*, 1990;**180**:50–76.
Garbarino J. Troubled youth, troubled families: the dynamics of adolescent maltreatment. In: Cicchetti D, Carlson V, eds. *Child maltreatment*. New York: Cambridge University Press, 1989:685–706.
Skuse D. Epidemiological and definitional issues in failure to thrive. In: Woolston J, ed. *Child and adolescent psychiatric clinics of North America*. Philadelphia: WB Saunders, 1993; 2(1): 37–59.
Skuse D, Bentovim A. Physical and emotional maltreatment. In: Rutter M, Taylor E, Hersov L, eds. *Child and adolescent psychiatry. Modern approaches*. 3rd ed. Oxford: Blackwell Scientific, 1994:209–29.

ABUSE AND SHORT STATURE

David Skuse, Jane Gilmour

Better is a dinner of herbs where love is than a
stalled ox and hatred therewith

Proverbs XV, 17

Many exceptionally short children with no
detectable organic disorder to account for their
condition fail to grow because they have been
subjected to longstanding abuse and neglect
within their families. Some such short children
have characteristic patterns of behaviour,
especially disorders of appetite, that should
draw attention to their predicament. The key
to the diagnosis is a good history. Failure to
recognise the aetiology of their condition may
imperil not only the children's future physical
development but also their intelligence, their
social adjustment, and their emotional
wellbeing. There are essentially two distinct
conditions of growth failure, unassociated with
organic disease, that are caused by abuse.
Appreciable numbers of children attending
specialist growth clinics suffer from one or
other of these frequently undiagnosed
disorders. The first we shall discuss, for which

no really satisfactory diagnostic label exists,
will be referred to as hyperphagic short stature
because of the associated insatiable appetite for
food and drink. It may be distinguished from
other cases of growth failure associated with
abuse in which affected children lose their
appetite. We have called the latter variant the
"anorexic subtype", which should not be
confused with anorexia nervosa for affected
children are not usually preoccupied with their
body image.

Developmental trends in abuse related growth failure

Impaired linear growth may follow failure to
thrive in infancy; recent prospective
longitudinal studies have shown that many
affected children remain significantly shorter
than their peers at least until puberty. Failure
to thrive is rarely due to overt abuse or
neglect. The usual cause is probably chronic
undernutrition. Children whose linear growth
is significantly retarded for that reason in the
first year or two of life do not usually show
much catch up growth subsequently, even if
their nutritional environment improves. They
are moderately short, usually 90–95% of
expected height for age. They show none of
the distinctive behavioural characteristics of
hyperphagic short stature, although they may
in due course become faddy or reluctant
eaters. Depending on the pattern of growth in
the period up to six months after birth, they
may also suffer from mild to moderately
impaired cognitive and psychomotor abilities.

Defining features of hyperphagic short stature

Hyperphagic short stature is not recognised
as a distinct entity within the International
Classification of Diseases, a deficiency which
hampers clinical recognition, inhibits
epidemiological investigations into prevalence,
and limits research into its aetiology and
management. Nevertheless, four key features
can be determined which together provide
compelling evidence for a diagnostic category:
firstly, a characteristic clinical picture
comprising symptoms, signs, and the results of
physiological tests; secondly, a common
aetiology; thirdly, a well recognised natural
history without intervention; and, fourthly, a
predictable favourable response to appropriate
management.

*Girl aged 8 years 2½ months
measuring 3' 4" (102 cm), a
height age of 4 years*

Children with hyperphagic short stature are not only exceptionally small for their age, they have a range of distinctive behavioural symptoms. The diagnosis is based on a combination of current and historical features. It is not normally made before 2 to 3 years, probably because the neuropsychological and neurophysiological mechanisms mediating the characteristic features require a certain maturation of the central nervous system to become evident. Symptoms include disorders of sleep and appetite, together with disturbed patterns of defecation or urination in many instances. The key aetiological factor is severe and prolonged stress, which is frequently but not exclusively associated with emotional abuse. There are, in our experience, some families whose children respond to stress in this way who use unusual and sadistic forms of physical and sexual maltreatment.

Most children living in stressful environments, however, do not display the characteristics of hyperphagic short stature. We suspect the key difference is that children who develop hyperphagic short stature have a genetic predisposition to do so. Our clinical and research experience suggests that about half the siblings in a family with an affected child who share both parents are at risk of developing the condition. Half siblings and step-siblings are at substantially lower risk. All children in a family with an affected sibling must be examined and a full history taken.

Anthropometry in hyperphagic short stature

Typically, the child's height for age is far below the third centile, between 85% and 90% of expected height for age. Growth is often at a low normal rate parallel to the centile line, although occasionally the condition presents with a variable and inconsistent growth trajectory. Weight for height is appropriate and head circumference is usually in proportion. Skinfold thickness and mid-upper arm circumference are usually normal. Parents are typically of average stature. In contrast, in the anorexia subtype of abuse related growth failure weight for height (or body mass index) is often below the 10th population centile.

Behavioural disturbance in hyperphagic short stature

Disorders of appetite and sleep

The most characteristic feature of this condition is hyperphagia or an insatiable appetite. Affected children do not behave like this because they are being starved by their parents. A long history of disordered behaviour with food is recounted, of which wandering around the home at night in search of it is typical. Parents respond to the child's hyperphagia by taking preventive action, placing locks on the bedroom, kitchen, and cupboard doors. Large quantities of food are often hoarded, usually in the child's room, in a way one consultant remarked was "like squirrels putting away nuts for the winter". Pica and the consumption of discarded food found in streets or wastebins can lead to gastrointestinal disturbance for which specialist opinion may be sought. Because of the child's propensity to "steal" food he or she may be fed separately from other family members. Teachers can often provide vivid accounts of disordered and bizarre behaviour at school dinner times. It is typical for parents to claim that if they let their children eat as much as they wanted they would gorge until they vomited and even, in a few cases, would not desist even at that point but would continue and consume their own vomit. Such behaviour resolves within a few days when the child is removed from stress and is not associated with any objective evidence of malnutrition.

Sleep is usually disrupted by nocturnal wanderings and, often, by nightmares. There may be an increase in active rapid eye movement (REM) sleep and a decrease in stages III and IV non-REM sleep relative to norms for the age group. Release of growth hormone is disrupted, although probably not directly as a consequence of the disturbed sleep pattern. Provocation tests of growth hormone production show a response which is abnormally low in most cases, providing the test is done while the child is still living in stressful conditions. A nocturnal profile of the pattern of growth hormone secretion shows diminished pulse amplitude, which has the

Growth curve of girl in figure on previous page related to events in her life. Her mother's height was 158 cm (25th centile) and her father's 178 cm (50th centile)

unique characteristic of recovery within a brief period in hospital. The abnormally low concentrations of growth hormone return to normal within a few weeks if the child is kept away from the stress or abuse. No other medical treatment is necessary in these cases.

Other behavioural features

Soiling may be an indicator of coincident sexual abuse. The usual story is not one of typical encopresis but comprises the following features. Firstly, it is persistent and frequent. Secondly, there are unusual patterns of associated behaviour—formed stools are concealed around the house and may even be found at school. Soiled clothing may also be disposed of in strange and devious ways, such as under carpets. Thirdly, faecal smearing is often reported, which, if it occurs principally in the child's bedroom, may indicate confinement for protracted periods.

Unusual patterns of urination are typical and may mislead the unwary by presenting as enuresis. Close questioning reveals the urination is as much over the bed as it is in it. The behaviour also occurs elsewhere in the house, behind cupboards, in fireplaces, in toy chests, and so on. There may be an exhibitionistic quality to the behaviour. It seems to be used primarily as an aggressive act. When sibling rivalry is a major component of family dysfunction urination occurs over the sibling's possessions.

Children with hyperphagic short stature have poor attention and may present with "hyperactivity". Invariably, there are associated learning difficulties. Poor receptive and expressive language skills are usual in combination with relatively less impaired non-verbal abilities. Affected children may be receiving special education on the grounds of mild to moderate learning difficulties. We are uncertain at present about the potential such children have for rapid and dramatic catch up cognitive growth when they are removed from their abusive environment. Most probably do not improve substantially.

Associated mood disturbance

Parents often complain their child had a difficult temperament from the earliest days, would not settle into routines, was irritable, and disliked close physical contact. Relationships with parents and siblings are typically marked by sullen withdrawal or defiant hostility. At home and at school an unhappy mood predominates and self esteem is poor. Antisocial behaviours may be habitual, especially petty pilfering at school. The objects taken are often virtually worthless (pens, rubbers, trinkets), and the behaviour seems to be a response to an emotional need. In younger children apparently senseless destructive acts (smashing new toys) are indicative of inner turmoil and distress.

Parental efforts at controlling undesirable behaviours are met with defiance; there is a seeming tolerance to most physical

punishments and, indeed, to physical pain and discomfort in general. Some parents resort to bizarre punitive methods, often with sadistic overtones—for example, shutting fingers in drawers, beating the soles of the feet, and making the child stand for prolonged periods with hands on head. Withdrawing food is a favourite technique for obvious reasons and probably serves to exacerbate the food related behaviour disorders.

Disorders of social relationships in cases of short stature related to abuse

In all cases of abuse related short stature no children with so poor a self image as these unhappy subjects could enjoy the reciprocity and mutual regard that typifies a true friendship. They wander around on the fringes of their peer group, drifting into casual liaisons with those who are similarly alienated, and consequently they are at high risk of becoming embroiled in antisocial activities. Relationships with adults are typified by sullen hostility and suspiciousness or, in some cases, by a promiscuous overfamiliarity which may have sexual undertones.

The depth of the alienation in family relationships may not be gauged by a casual observer in the surgery or outpatient clinic. Abused children may nevertheless be brought for medical attention and investigations. A hint of the degree to which they are regarded with contempt by their caretakers may be gathered from remarks made in your presence—for example, a father telling his 8 year old son "You've got custard for brains". Children with this condition often have an anxious attachment to their abusive parents and so will be very reluctant to separate from them. They may even be warned in your presence not to tell "porky pies". Faced with a profound fear of retribution on revealing the truth of their predicament, many children with abuse related short stature will simply prefer to remain mute.

Management

When a diagnosis of emotional abuse leading to a delay in growth is suspected a coordinated response with the local social services department is necessary. A case conference will be held, and the services of other experts such as a child psychiatrist and paediatric endocrinologist may be deemed necessary. Protection from further abuse should be the first priority, and this will usually mean removing the child from the abusive environment. Sometimes it is possible to persuade the parents to give up the child voluntarily. In most cases legal proceedings must be instituted, and there are three main sources of evidence which will serve as the basis for a successful intervention. Firstly, there is the evidence of the associated abuse. While emotional abuse as such is notoriously difficult to prove, a history of sexual abuse or physical abuse, or both, may be obtained together with associated physical signs.

Diagnostic criteria for hyperphagic short stature

These features must be present:
- Height for age below third population centile with growth failure
- Body mass index in normal range
- Age greater than 2 years

At least one of these symptoms must be present and should reflect a current pattern of behaviour:
- Steals food at home or school, or both
- Gorges and vomits

Two of these symptoms must be present and should reflect a persistent pattern of behaviour:
- Eats excessively
- Polydipsia
- Hoards food
- Wakes at night and searches for food
- Forages for discarded food or rummages for food in bins

Secondly, growth hormone provocation tests should be done before a hospital admission and again after three weeks in hospital or foster care. In hyperphagic cases reversibility from insufficiency to normal or even supranormal concentrations may be demonstrated over this brief period. In anorexic subtypes the initial growth hormone concentrations are usually high to normal and do not show significant change when the child is removed from stress. In such cases repeated testing is unnecessary. There may be documented evidence that the affected child has shown catch up linear growth during a prolonged period in hospital or a former period of foster care. Thirdly, there may be evidence of a deterioration over time in cognitive abilities while the child is living in the abusive home. Motor development will in general be less affected than skills based on language such as practical reasoning. Serial testing every six months or so with a standardised instrument such as the Griffith's scales can yield valuable information. Scores should be calculated as a percentage, with the quotient of mental age divided by chronological age used to view trends.

Natural history

Absolutely characteristic of the hyperphagic short stature syndrome is a dramatic increase in the children's velocity of linear growth once they have been removed from their abusive environment. It is not unusual to find a sixfold to tenfold increase within a few months. Mental development may also increase provided an appropriate attachment is established between the child and the carer and the child is encouraged to learn in a comparatively structured and stimulating environment. Poor attention is a feature of the syndrome and militates against efficient learning. If bizarre patterns of behaviour persist for longer than a few months once the child is settled into a stable new home the question of whether the child is now being abused by his or her new carers must be faced.

Should the child be returned home a diminution in growth rate will ensue. Unwary doctors may erroneously conclude that the potential for growth has now been fulfilled, especially if the subsequent trajectory is parallel to the centile lines. Consider the growth curve on page 35, which is the growth record of the girl shown on page 34. Rapid increases in height during her admission to hospital and at boarding school were followed by stable linear growth. When she was 15 she ran away from home and her height eventually reached the 25th centile. The potential for catch up growth is substantially greater in cases of hyperphagic short stature such as this (where the growth failure was associated with emotional abuse) than in the anorexic subtype of abuse related short stature. Both are associated with disorders of appetite, but the hyperphagia rapidly resolves when the child is removed from stress whereas an anorexic pattern of appetite disturbance tends to persist and recovery in terms of height for age is much slower and less complete.

Further reading
Skuse D, Albanese A, Stanhope R, *et al*. A new stress-related syndrome of growth failure and hyperphagia in children, associated with reversibility of growth-hormone insufficiency. *Lancet* 1996;**348**:353–8.
Skuse D. The relationship between deprivation, physical growth and the impaired development of language. In: Fletcher P, ed. *Specific speech and language disorders in children*. London: Whurr Publications, 1992:29–50.
Skuse DH, Gill D, Reilly S, *et al*. Failure to thrive and the risk of child abuse: a prospective population survey. *J Med Screening* 1995;**2**:145–50.
Skuse D, Pickles A, Wolke D, *et al*. Postnatal growth and mental development: evidence for a 'sensitive period'. *J Child Psychol Psychiatry* 1994;**35**:521–45.

CHILD SEXUAL ABUSE–I

Frank Bamford, Raine Roberts

What is child sexual abuse?

Child sexual abuse is any use of children for the sexual gratification of adults.

Who abuses and who is abused?

The abuser is almost always a male known to the child: a relative (father, grandfather, uncle, or older brother); a member of the household (stepfather or mother's cohabitants); or a temporary carer—for example, teenage male babysitters. Note that abusing men may move after the discovery of abuse to another household of similar composition. A few cases occur in the context of organised abuse (page 52).

Child sexual abuse may occur in any part of society but is discovered more commonly in poor families.

Children of all ages and either sex may be sexually abused.

What happens?

Sexual abuse entails all types of sexual activity, often with escalating intrusiveness.

Children may be exposed to indecent acts, pornographic photography, or external genital contact in the form of being fondled, masturbating an adult, or being used for intercrural intercourse. Finally, they may be penetrated orally, vaginally, or anally.

How often does sexual abuse occur?

Nobody knows how often sexual abuse occurs. It is certain that a lot of abuse is undiagnosed and equally certain that false diagnoses may be catastrophic.

Five main risk factors predispose to child sexual abuse:

- Previous incest or sexual deviance in the family
- New male member of the household with a record of sexual offences
- Loss of inhibition due to alcohol
- Loss of maternal libido or sexual rejection of father
- A paedophilic sexual orientation, especially in relation to sex rings and pornography.

Do children tell?

Sometimes children tell other people, but many are threatened to stop them telling. They may receive compensatory treats or presents.

Disclosure after a long period of abuse is common and may be followed by retraction. The statements of young children about sexual abuse should be taken seriously and, if possible, written down verbatim. Repeated questioning is potentially harmful and may evoke less truthful answers. Care is needed in understanding exactly what the child is saying—for example, "Daddy hurt my bum" may be interpreted in several ways, whereas "Daddy put his willie in my mouth" can hardly be anything other than abuse.

Does the non-abusing parent tell?

Sometimes the parent who is not sexually abusing the child will tell someone about the abuse, but collusion within families may occur, as in physical abuse. Beware of allegations made by parents in disputes about access or custody. Do not dismiss them but treat them with great caution.

How may sexual abuse present?

Sexual abuse may present in several ways:

- Statements of the child
- Symptoms due to local trauma or infection—for example, perineal soreness, vaginal discharge, and anal pain or bleeding
- Symptoms attributable to emotional effects—for example, loss of concentration, enuresis, encopresis, anorexia, and parasuicide. A change in behaviour is important
- Sexualised conduct or inappropriate sexual knowledge for young children. Remember that such conduct or knowledge may be derived from observing others or from pornographic videos, but if a child describes pain or the quality of semen, physical interference is probable.

What should be recorded?

Doctors dealing with child sexual abuse should keep a record of who asked them to see the child, who accompanied him or her, who raised the question of sexual abuse, who gave the history, and who was present at the examination.

The history should include details of the incident(s) causing suspicion; a full paediatric history, with particular emphasis on genitourinary or bowel symptoms; and details of previous abuse or sexual offences within the family or household.

Should the child be examined and where?

The child should be examined but not without the knowledge and agreement of a parent (or the order of a court). Mothers of preadolescent children should always be invited to be present, except in the most exceptional circumstances. Adolescent patients should be asked whether they wish a parent to be present.

It is usually counterproductive to examine a resistant child, and if his or her cooperation cannot be obtained the examination should be deferred unless there are urgent medical reasons to proceed.

The child should be examined as soon as optimal arrangements can be made. Few children require urgent examination, but healing of signs may occur within a few days and examination should not be delayed by other inquiries.

Repetitive examination is usually abusive and should be avoided unless it is necessary for therapeutic purposes or when there are reasonable grounds for believing that there is ongoing abuse.

The examination should be conducted in absolute privacy and in an environment where the child can be comfortable—not behind screens in open wards or in police stations.

There should be adequate equipment for any necessary diagnostic tests. Recording and photographic facilities are an advantage but their value is outweighed if they cause distress to the child or mean that another examination has to be conducted.

Some centres now have colposcopes. They provide good illuminaton and magnification and enable a standard photographic record of the findings to be made. Where such facilities are available the need for re-examination of children for legal purposes can usually be avoided.

Consent for examination

Usually consent for examination should be obtained from a parent or a person with parental responsibility. When a child is the subject of court proceedings the consent of the court is required. Under the *Children Act 1989* children of sufficient understanding to make an informed decision have a right to refuse examination.

If a doctor is consulted by a parent who alleges child sexual abuse, consent to examination of the child is implied and failure to examine may be regarded as negligent. Likewise examination of the genitalia or anus would be expected if there was a complaint of relevant symptoms.

Who should examine?

A person with skill in paediatric examination who is familiar with normal genital and anal appearances of children should conduct the examination. When physical abnormalities are expected from the history a forensic physician should be invited to examine or to be present during the examination so that it need not be repeated and a second opinion is available in doubtful cases.

Who should be present?

The only people present at the examination should be the child, his or her parent, and the examiner(s)—no one else—except, with the agreement of the parents, an occasional observer in training.

What about acute sexual abuse?

When abuse is thought to have been recent (within 6 days) or there is serious genital injury forensic evidence should not be compromised. Examination should be deferred, if consistent with safety, until a forensic physician can be present. Nobody should remove clothing or attempt to clean or bath the child. Junior medical staff should not examine suspected victims unless the child urgently needs medical attention.

CHILD SEXUAL ABUSE–II

Frank Bamford, Raine Roberts

In child sexual abuse genital and anal examination should be in the context of a general clinical examination and include a search for other forms of abuse and an appraisal of growth, development, and health. The behaviour of the child in the presence of his or her parent should be noted.

Why should the genitalia be examined?

The genitalia should be examined in child sexual abuse for five main reasons:

- To detect traumatic or infective conditions that may require treatment
- To evaluate the nature of any abuse. Normal genital and anal appearances do not exclude the diagnosis, but in young children they make penetrative abuse unlikely
- To provide forensic evidence that may be helpful to the future protection of children
- To reassure the child, who sometimes feels that serious damage has been done
- To start the process of recovery.

How to examine the genitalia and anus

Cooperation during an examination is best achieved by telling children exactly what is happening and allowing them to feel in control by asking them to help. Let them take the swabs if they wish. The child may lie on her back for vulval inspection or on her side as for anal examination. Some children prefer to be examined in the knee to chest position, face downwards on the couch. In this position the important posterior edge of the hymen is often more clearly visualised than in the frog leg supine position, and the use of a moistened swab or glass rod to examine the edge of the hymen can be avoided. With children up to 7 years old it is sometimes better for them to lie along the length of their mother's knee, facing forwards, with the mother gently flexing and abducting the hips. Adequate inspection requires a relaxed child, and the child should be allowed to choose the position of the examination.

Should fingers or a speculum be inserted?

Some doctors insert a finger to assess the tone of the anal sphincter but generally it should be avoided. Views differ as to its importance. In rare cases of violent anal assault proctoscopy is likely to yield more information.

In a small number of cases in which vaginal examination or repair is necessary the child should be given a general anaesthetic. General anaesthesia should also be considered if there is vaginal bleeding after suspected abuse.

Can sexual abuse be proved by clinical examination?

Semen or blood of a group different from that of the child would, if present within the vagina or rectum or on the perineum in a prepubertal child, be conclusive evidence of interference, but such cases are uncommon in forensic practice and wholly exceptional in paediatric practice. Lubricants or hairs are of similar importance. Genital infection with *Neisseria gonorrhoeae* is indicative of contact with an infected person in 98% of cases, but all other findings can be produced by circumstances or conditions other than sexual abuse. It follows that, with the exceptions mentioned, the concept of a single, conclusive diagnostic sign is invalid.

How patent is a child's vagina?

The likelihood or otherwise of penetration may be inferred from the size of the hymenal orifice, but it cannot be used as a sole basis for the diagnosis of abuse. Individual hymens vary substantially from the imperforate to the congenitally almost absent, and the hymen may occasionally be cribriform. In most prepubescent children it is a membrane with a circular or crescentic opening and a smooth, regular margin that may be either thin or rounded.

The diameter is difficult to measure accurately, but in most young children, except those approaching puberty, the unstretched hymenal orifice is no more than 0·5–0·6 cm, increasing slightly as puberty approaches. Rarely, the size of the hymenal orifice may be greater but a transverse hymenal diameter of 1·5 cm in association with other evidence of trauma would be highly suggestive of abuse. The hymen is a fairly elastic membrane but as the diameter of an adult index finger is about 1·5 cm and that of an erect penis two or three times greater, penetration is very unlikely to have occurred if there is an intact, unstretched hymen.

It is important to spend some time carefully observing the hymen without coming to any conclusion about it. A hymen appearing undamaged will sometimes open up as the child relaxes and tears and bumps may be seen. Gentle traction of the labia majora

Right: Tear of hymen, left lateral, would have been missed without use of Glaister's rod

forwards and downwards may help to display the hymen more clearly and will make the orifice appear larger. Measurements with and without traction together with a diagram of the shape of the hymenal orifice should be recorded.

What causes irregularity or tearing of the hymen?

The hymen may be damaged in four main ways:

- By sexual abuse
- By genital disease. A careful history is important
- By self injury. This is unusual because it is painful, but damage to the hymen may occur by the insertion of foreign bodies
- By accidental injury. This is also unusual because after infancy the introitus is protected by the labia.

Below left: Be careful not to mistake vestibule for hymen. On left vestibule is seen while middle picture (closer picture of same child) shows red crescent of hymen

Far right: Lichen sclerosus et atrophicus. Characteristic depigmentation of the labia majora extending to the anus. (Commonly there is wrinkling of the skin of the labia, from atrophy, and sometimes bruising or bleeding)

Petechial bruising on palate. Always look in mouth for signs of oral sex

Note that the hymen adjacent to the urethra may have a notched apearance and it is important to distinguish this from hymenal injury.

Signs of intercrural intercourse

There are usually no signs of intercrural intercourse but occasionally bruising of the perineum may occur. It may cause patchy redness on the labia and perineum, but this is common in other conditions—for example, enuresis and poor hygiene. The rounded labial contour may be flattened, but it is not a reliable sign as flattening can be due to tight clothing. There may be a split of the posterior fourchette and a subsequent scar. Finally, the pressure of a penis against the hymen may stretch it and the child may think that there has been penetration.

Signs of buggery

The signs of buggery are likely to be most prominent in young children. In many cases there are no abnormal signs but look for evidence of external trauma, skin changes, and anal dilatation.

External trauma in anal abuse

Superficial fissures are common in children and may be caused by overstretching of the anus. They may be seen in abused as well as non-abused childen. Of greater importance in relation to abuse are deep fissures crossing the anal skin margin. Scars or anal skin tags may be left but not in all cases. Be careful to distinguish fissures from prominent folds in the anal canal.

Swelling of the skin around the anal verge may be seen occasionally after recent abuse and thickening after repeated abuse. The skin of the anal verge may become rounded and smooth. Distinguish from lichen sclerosus et atrophicus, perianal moniliasis, and scratching by children infected with threadworms. Skin changes by themselves are not sufficient to lead to investigation of abuse.

Perineal bruising or bleeding without reasonable explanation raises substantial suspicion. It must be distinguished from haemangiomata and dilated vessels. Veins may be dilated in association with bowel disorder.

Warts around the anus (or vaginal introitus) may be transmitted by genital contact. They are strongly suggestive of sexual abuse, especially if a wart virus of a genitally transmitted type is identified. Genital warts are usually smaller than common warts and appear as multiple papules along the inner surface of the labia or circumferentially around the anus. They occur particularly where skin is moist. Parents or children who have common warts on their hands may infect skin in the region of the genitalia or anus during toileting.

Anal dilatation

Given that the bowel is normal and that the child does not suffer from any neurological disorder, abnormal patency is indicative of something hard and large having passed through the anus, but it is impossible to be sure whether the object has passed upwards or come downwards. A history of bowel problems or of medical investigation or treatment is therefore important. "Reflex" anal dilatation is not a true reflex. It amounts to relaxation of the anal sphincter about 10 seconds after the anus has been inspected so that an initially closed anus opens during the course of examination (alternatively an anus open at first closes during the examination and then opens again).

VARIATIONS IN HYMEN

Right: Two holes in hymen

Far right top: Septate hymen. Bands are usually vertical. Hymenal tags (not shown) may be incomplete bands and be mistaken for tears

Far right below: Bump on hymen. Hymen has probably been torn posteriorly leaving bumps and slight thickening

CLASSIC INJURY OF ATTEMPTED PENILE PENETRATION

Right: Haematoma of hymen and split of posterior fourchette

Far right: Recently torn hymen in teenage girl. Hymen usually tears in posterior half

Inflamed, thickened hymen, in this case caused by rubbing

Redness caused by rubbing

Anal closure and continence is dependent upon the internal anal sphincter. If it is incompetent because of stretching or injury there is likely to be soiling. The internal anal sphincter may be relaxed physiologically by faeces in the lower rectum. In examining children in whom abuse is suspected it is important to ensure that they are relaxed, that the rectum is empty, and that there is no other source of pressure on it. When the internal sphincter is incompetent the external sphincter may be able to maintain closure for a short time but cannot sustain it, hence the changes seen during examination. "Reflex" anal dilatation may be a pointer to sexual abuse but is not reliable as a sole diagnostic sign and its significance is currently unproved.

Should tests be done for sexually transmitted disease?

Sexually transmitted disease should always be tested for in children molested by strangers. In intrafamilial cases obtain swabs unless it is clearly going to cause distress. Sometimes it is helpful to get suspected abusing parents to attend a genitourinary medicine clinic.

Taking a low vaginal swab at the initial examination may enable a presumptive diagnosis of gonorrhoea by Gram staining of a smear, but definitive diagnosis depends on culture and selective tests. If contact has been recent, a repeat swab will be needed because the incubation period of gonorrhoea is two to seven days. Swabs should also be taken from the pharynx and rectum.

Chlamydia trachomatis may cause asymptomatic infection. It can be detected by culture but this is not always available. If available special swabs and transport medium should be used. Enzyme immunoassay and direct immunofluorescent antibody tests are available but have not been fully evaluated in children. Interpretation of positive cultures in young children is difficult because perinatally acquired infection may persist for two or more years.

If herpetic lesions are seen on the genitalia the base of a lesion should be rubbed with a swab which should then be placed in virus transport medium for subsequent culture. Specimens can be stored at 4°C if any delay is anticipated. Typing techniques may enable matching with samples from a suspected abuser.

Trichomonas vaginalis is very uncommon in prepubertal children after the neonatal period because of vaginal alkalinity. It may survive in a prepubertal vagina for a very short period, and its presence is indicative of recent sexual abuse. After puberty it often causes vulvovaginitis but it may be asymptomatic. Non-sexual transmission is uncommon. Diagnosis is made by observation of mobile flagellate organisms on microscopic examination of vaginal secretion in a drop of physiological saline and by culture with appropriate media.

ANAL DILATATION

Right: Place hands gently on buttocks and wait

Far right: Both sphincters open. Do not pull with fingers as false positive results will occur. Ensure rectum is empty. (Note that faeces can be seen in this girl's rectum)

Child sexual abuse–II

Buggery: Top pictures show swelling, bruising, and fissures of anal margin caused by recent buggery

Right: Anal dilatation, bruising, and fissure

Far right: Appearance of healed anus 10 days later

It is now very uncommon in Britain to see children with clinical signs of syphilis. The infection is excluded by appropriate serological tests immediately and three months after the last possible abusive contact.

Tests for antibodies to HIV and hepatitis B may be required later in specific cases, as may pregnancy tests in post-pubertal girls.

Medical management

The medical management of child sexual abuse is part of an interdisciplinary process. Communication with other agencies is essential.

Preliminary consultation

"Where uncertainty exists doctors will often find it helpful to test out professional hypotheses before initial concerns about child abuse are shared with non-medical colleagues. Doctors should clarify their own thoughts about a particular case, and with advice as

appropriate from senior or more senior colleagues, reach a critical threshold of professional concern. When a critical threshold of concern is reached doctors must be prepared to share these concerns with the statutory agencies for further evaluation and discussion **within a time frame which is not detrimental to the child's interests**" (*Child Protection: Medical Responsibilities*, Department of Health, British Medical Association, Conference of Medical Royal Colleges).

Possible sexual abuse

- If child sexual abuse is only a possibility—for example, the child has made a vague statement, there are behavioural changes, vulval or anal soreness, or family risk factors—take a careful history from the carer and write down anything said by the child but do not engage in an intrusive interview.
- If the history points to a probability of abuse refer the child to an experienced person.

*Genital and anal findings which **may** indicate abuse*

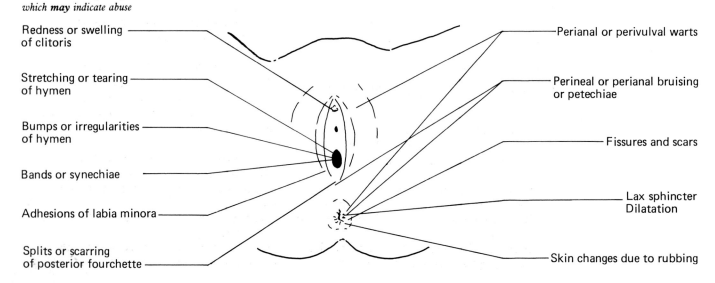

Redness or swelling of clitoris

Stretching or tearing of hymen

Bumps or irregularities of hymen

Bands or synechiae

Adhesions of labia minora

Splits or scarring of posterior fourchette

Perianal or perivulval warts

Perineal or perianal bruising or petechiae

Fissures and scars

Lax sphincter Dilatation

Skin changes due to rubbing

Treatment of cases of child sexual abuse by primary care doctors

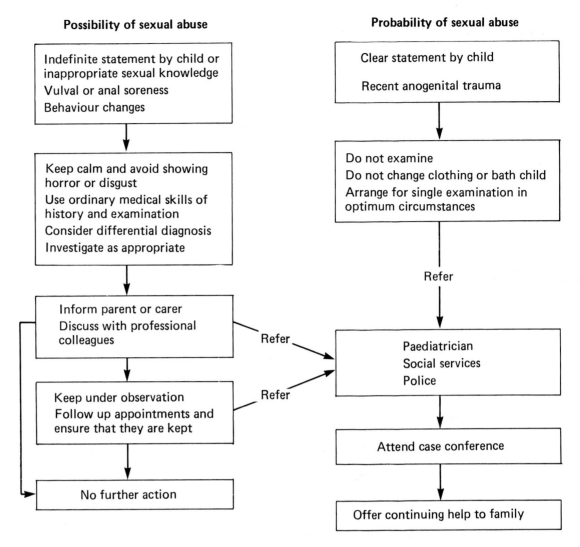

Possibility of sexual abuse

Indefinite statement by child or inappropriate sexual knowledge
Vulval or anal soreness
Behaviour changes

Keep calm and avoid showing horror or disgust
Use ordinary medical skills of history and examination
Consider differential diagnosis
Investigate as appropriate

Inform parent or carer
Discuss with professional colleagues

Keep under observation
Follow up appointments and ensure that they are kept

No further action

Probability of sexual abuse

Clear statement by child

Recent anogenital trauma

Do not examine
Do not change clothing or bath child
Arrange for single examination in optimum circumstances

Refer

Paediatrician
Social services
Police

Attend case conference

Offer continuing help to family

Refer

Refer

● If the history is not clearly indicative of abuse examine the whole child, including the genitalia, and take swabs if appropriate.
● Discuss the case with colleagues in the practice, including health visitors and possibly school nurses. Hospital doctors should discuss the case with the family's general practitioner. Some regions have experienced staff who are willing to advise. Ascertain whether the family is known by or has caused concern to the social services.
● Tell the carer of your findings and opinion.
● Arrange follow up visits and ensure that appointments are kept.

Probable sexual abuse
● If child sexual abuse is probable because of a clear statement from the child or unexplained recent vaginal or anal injury inform the police and social services department promptly, with the knowledge and, if possible, the agreement of the carer.
● Do not examine the child—arrange for a full, single paediatric and forensic examination at which suitable samples and photographs can be obtained.
● Check that the medical welfare of the child has been safeguarded—that is, infections

treated and, if appropriate, pregnancy tests and postcoital contraception provided.
● Facilitate interviews of the child by a psychiatrist, psychologist, police officer, or social worker agreed by all the parties concerned. Avoid further abuse of the child by preventing different people going over the same material repetitively.
● Ascertain whether there are other children at risk and arrange to examine them.
● Participate in a multidisciplinary case conference.
● Ensure long term follow up with child psychiatrists as appropriate.

Allegations by an adult against another
   When an adult accuses another adult of child sexual abuse refer the case to an experienced person because such cases often lead to litigation.

Violent sexual assault outside the family
   Refer all cases in which children are violently assaulted outside the family to the police.
   Do not touch or examine the child, except in an emergency.
   Ensure the medical welfare of the child as in other cases but after forensic examinations are

complete. Almost all victims require skilled psychiatric help.

Confidentiality

The overriding duty is to the child. "There is no law of confidentiality which would command silence when the welfare of the child is concerned". It is usually possible to obtain the consent of one parent to examination and disclosure—in any event you are obliged to make sure that the parent(s) understand that information will be shared. Be careful not to make promises of secrecy.

Further reading

Bays J, Chadwick D. Medical diagnosis of the sexuality abused child. *Child Abuse Negl* 1993;**17**:91–110.

Berenson AB. A longitudinal study of hymenal morphology in the first 3 years of life. *Pediatrics* 1995;**4**:490–6.

De Jong A, Finkel MA. Sexual abuse of children. *Curr Probl Paediatrics* 1990;**20**:489–567.

Department of Health and Social Security. *Diagnosis of child sexual abuse: guidance for doctors*. London: HMSO, 1988.

Home Office, Department of Health, Department of Education and Science, Welsh Office. *Working together under the Children Act 1989*. London: HMSO, 1991.

Kerns DI, Ritter ML, Concave hymenal variations in suspected child abuse victims. *Pediatrics* 1992;**90**:265–72.

Royal College of Physicians. *Physical signs of sexual abuse in children*. London: Royal College of Physicians, 1996.

MUNCHAUSEN SYNDROME BY PROXY

Roy Meadow

RAISING THE COLLEGE OF PHYSICIANS

Baron von Munchausen, born in 1720, was a German mercenary and a gifted raconteur. Richard Asher in 1951 dedicated Munchausen syndrome to the memory of the baron because the patients had his characteristic of travelling widely and telling false stories.

The picture shows Baron von Munchausen raising the College of Physicians of London into the air for three months (during which the health of its patients was never better)

The term Munchausen's syndrome is applied to adults who present themselves to doctors and to hospitals with false stories of illness, so causing themselves to have needless admissions and investigations. Munchausen syndrome by proxy was used first in 1977 to describe child abuse caused by mothers who present their children to doctors and hospitals with false stories of illness and by substantiating the stories by fabricating physical signs. Abuse results partly from the direct actions of the mother—for example, giving drugs to make the child unconscious—and partly from the doctors, who arrange investigations, hospital admissions, or needless treatments for the child at the mother's instigation. The term is best used as a description of a type of child abuse rather than to imply that the perpetrator is "suffering from Munchausen syndrome by proxy". Though many of the perpetrators share personality traits, they are not a homogeneous group and different perpetrators abuse children for different reasons.

Increasing recognition of Munchausen syndrome by proxy abuse (synonyms: factitious illness by proxy, Meadow's syndrome) has led to many cases of non-accidental poisoning (page 24) and smothering (page 28) coming to light. Most of these are happening in the context of repetitive false illnesses, but when poisoning or smothering is isolated it is unwise to use the term Munchausen syndrome by proxy. Moreover, in all cases of child abuse it is more important to define the nature and the extent of the abuse and the risks for the child rather than worry about terminology.

Definition

In relation to children the term may be used if:

● Physical or psychological symptoms or signs are intentionally produced or invented by a parent or other carer
● The perpetrator, at least initially, denies inventing or causing the symptoms or signs
● The symptoms and signs diminish or cease when the child is separated from the perpetrator.

There is a case for including motivation in the diagnostic criteria in that the perpetrator's usual motive is to satisfy personal needs ranging from assuming the sick role by proxy to other ways of gaining sympathy and attention for themselves. Although there may be secondary economic gain for the perpetrator in terms of disability of other benefits, such external incentives are not the prime reason for the abuse.

Factitious illness

There are different stages of falsification and, although there may be escalation from the first to the third, each alone may be very harmful to the child.

False illness story alone—Even though the mother is not directly harming her child, the child may suffer considerably. False illness story alone may cause a child to undergo many needless investigations and treatments as well as restriction of activity and education.

False illness story plus fabrication of signs—The mother in addition to the false story seeks to convince doctors by tampering with the child's samples or medical records.

Induced illness—The false story is substantiated by poisoning, smothering, or other physical injury which causes genuine illness. This third stage is less common than the other two, but it features more prominently in child care and criminal proceedings because of the strength of the evidence, which may include detailed toxicology, video recordings, and other robust forensic evidence.

Clinical features

Young preschool children are the main victims. The abuse usually starts in the first year of life, often within the first month (and sometimes even earlier, for unusual events in pregnancy are common). It is uncommon after the age of 5 years and probably involves a degree of awareness or complicity by the older child for the false illness to continue to deceive doctors. Boys and girls are equally affected. About half the siblings of an index child suffer from either similar or another form of abuse. There is an increased incidence of unexpected death of previous children.

Epidemiology

A two year survey of Munchausen syndrome by proxy in the United Kingdom suggested that the annual incidence for children under the age of 1 is at least 3 per 100 000.

Munchausen syndrome by proxy

Presentation

The child is usually presented with problems relating to one system—for instance recurrent seizures or a story of diarrhoea and vomiting. A minority present as if they have a multisystem disorder. Some of the children will have genuine illness in addition to the superimposed illness—thus a child may have occasional genuine seizures but be presented as having many seizures each day. A whole range of physical signs are fabricated.

Usually the illness story is presented consistently by the mother and the periodic events of illness start only in her presence. The father may be unusually absent from visits to outpatient clinics or the ward. While some mothers are model parents in terms of keeping appointments and complying with treatment, it is quite common to find a paradoxical mixture of pleading for more treatment and investigation on the one hand and failure to attend for such tests and appointments on the other (presumably because the mother knows they are not needed). Compliance with treatment may be chaotic: though apnoea alarms are given out they are not used appropriately, and anticonvulsants which are prescribed are not given for a period and then given in excess. Unusual failure of equipment is common, with lines becoming disconnected or infected and catheters breaking.

The mothers usually stay with one general practitioner and, when referred to hospital, with one specialist. The child's referral to other specialists is made by the general practitioner or specialist, and the child may be transferred from one centre of excellence to another; repetitive investigation results.

Common presentations

Nervous system	Seizures, apnoea, drowsiness
Gastrointestinal	Vomiting, diarrhoea, failure to thrive
Respiratory	Apnoea, breathlessness
Renal	Haematuria
Endocrine	Glycosuria, hypernatraemia, biochemical abnormality
Allergy	Rashes, diarrhoea, vomiting, fever

Less common presentations

Otorhinolaryngological	Chronic otitis
Educational	Dyslexia, disability, special needs
Skin	Dermatitis artefacta, abscesses
Orthopaedic	Locked joints
Haematological	Anaemia
Cardiovascular	Sick sinus syndrome, arrhythmias, syncope
Child abuse	False allegations of sexual or physical abuse

Factitious signs

Sign	Cause
Bleeding	Haematemesis, haemoptysis, haematuria, or other bleeding. Usually the mother uses her own blood, either by self injury or from a vaginal tampon
Seizures	Hypoxia (smothering), drugs
Failure to thrive	Withholding or diluting food, sucking back feed from stomach with a nasogastric tube
Diarrhoea	Laxatives
Vomiting	Emetics, fingers pushed down child's throat, or mother presents own vomit as child's
Fevers	Falsifying chart or heating thermometer
Dermatitis	Caustic solutions or scratching/injuring skin
Chronic discharge	From ears, vagina, anus by repetitive poking with small object
Anaemia	By venepuncture or disconnecting intravenous line to drain blood
Endocrine abnormality	Addition of drug or chemical to child's urine or blood sample
Hypertension	Altering entries on blood pressure charts or instructions concerning size of cuff to be used for measurement
Faeculant vomits	Vomiting is induced and then faeces are stirred into the bowl of vomit

Consequences

- Repetitive, unpleasant or dangerous investigations and treatments
- Induced illness as a result of the mother's actions (for example, from injection of contaminated solutions into intravenous lines)
- Chronic invalidism as a result of the child being indoctrinated with the concept of being ill
- Abnormal illness behaviour when the child grows up (sometimes amounting to Munchausen's syndrome) as a result of being encouraged and taught to participate in the deception of doctors.

Perpetrator

In over 90% of cases the perpetrator is the child's natural mother. In 5% of cases it is another female carer, and in less than 5% it is the child's father. It is most unusual for there to be collusion between mother and father; the innocent partner is usually completely unaware and dumbfounded by the deception.

Commonly the perpetrating mother has incurred emotional abuse as a child, particularly in terms of lack of love and respect from her own mother. Women with a nursing background are overrepresented among the perpetrators. Previous encounters with a psychiatrist are common, but it is rare for the mother to have mental illness identified. Most of them do have personality disorders, however, and a minority have somatising disorders to such an extent that they may be labelled as suffering from Munchausen's syndrome. The male perpetrators are similar to the female though with a predominance of histrionic personality characteristics.

Some of the mothers are hospital addicts, who seem to relish a good paediatric unit. They form close relationships with the staff and take the lead in fund raising. Other perpetrators, however, behave more like the usual parents who abuse children, being reluctant to visit their child in hospital, and being over-ready to complain or be litigious about medical care.

Many mothers achieve considerable self respect from their role in caring for an "ill" child and cherish their close relationship with doctors, nurses and support agencies, while others gain sympathy within their family and their communities (as a result of seeking publicity), as well as support from parents of other sick children. For some the motive seems to be to reclaim an absent husband. There is a minority, however, in which resentment and violence feature high in the motivation—the mother resenting the impact of the baby on her life or being unable to tolerate the problems of caring for a difficult child.

Warning signals

In addition to the general features in the box there are particular groups of children who are more likely to include some with factitious illness: these include those receiving intensive treatment for severe allergy, recurrent apnoea, or sleep apnoea, those receiving prolonged parenteral feeding; and children incurring Nissen fundoplication for gastro-oesophageal reflux.

Warning signals

Illness
- Unexplained and prolonged
- Very rare

Symptoms and signs
- Incongruous
- Only when mother present
- Allergy

Mother
- Hospital addict
- Not too worried
- Publicity seeking

Father
- Uninvolved with child's "illness"

Treatment
- Ineffective
- Not tolerated

Family
- Previous child death
- Child abuse
- Multiple illness

Pets
- Sudden death
- Unusual illnesses

Action and reaction

Extreme fabricated illness is very serious and may be life threatening, requiring immediate liaison with social services and the police to protect the child. It is important not to overreact, however, just because a mother is lying or fabricating signs. Sometimes a mother may add blood to her child's urine or alter a temperature chart to dissuade the doctors from discharging her child from hospital before she is sufficiently reassured and ready to cope at home. Such minor events are common and should be sorted out sympathetically and promptly in a way that dissuades the mother from giving false illness stories or fabricating signs again. Other mothers perceive or exaggerate their child's symptoms because of anxiety and stress.

Usually the diagnosis is a paediatric one. An experienced paediatrician is needed to decide whether the child's symptoms and signs are the results of natural illness or are false. In a minority of cases—for instance, fictitious sexual abuse or imposed psychological symptoms—another specialist such as a child psychiatrist or child psychologist may be the most appropriate person to make the diagnosis.

Establishing that the illness is factitious can be difficult and requires much resourcefulness. Verification of the alleged illness events should be sought from other family members. Contact with the general practitioner and health visitor are important, and their records can be checked against the hospital records for consistency of illness events. Every opportunity should be taken to acquire forensic evidence by way of toxicological evidence or testing to determine the origin of blood in a sample or on clothing.* A period of observation in hospital, without parental visiting, can be a much kinder and more useful diagnostic test for the child than yet more invasive investigation.

The long term outcome for children who have been abused by fictitious illness is worrying. There is a significant incidence of recurrence of abuse of children who remain in maternal care and significant morbidity in the long term, suggesting that Munchausen syndrome by proxy abuse reflects a serious disorder of the mother–child relationship and the chance of long lasting harm.

Not quite Munchausen syndrome by proxy

There are times when severe Munchausen syndrome by proxy abuse seems to be an extension of commonplace parental behaviour concerning their child's health. Each of the types of parental behaviour listed below is well recognised and not rare. Although they may be disadvantageous to the child and sometimes harmful, most of the time the behaviour is contained by appropriate medical help and counselling. In some circumstances, however, each of these behaviour patterns may be a cause of serious child abuse and may necessitate child protection procedures. When

A 6 year old boy had nine colonoscopies, a bronchoscopy, gastroscopy, two jejunal biopsies, and angiography. He incurred a Nissen fundoplication and an ileostomy and lived on total parental nutrition for four years. The mother did not harm him directly, she merely presented a false story about his intractable vomiting and diarrhoea. After separation from his mother the child fed normally and became healthy.

that is necessary it is unwise to invoke the term Munchausen syndrome by proxy and better merely to deal with the way in which the child is at risk or suffering as a result of the parents actions.

Over anxious parents—whose extreme anxiety communicates itself to the child, thereby perpetuating and enhancing adverse behaviour or ill health. Some mothers perceive symptoms out of fearfulness or exaggerate them to impress doctors. Impatient doctors compound the problem.

Doctor shopping—For a parent to seek a second or third opinion about their child may be sensible, but an eighth or ninth further opinion is likely to be abusive in terms of repeated investigation and needless treatment.

False allegations of paternal abuse in the context of custody disputes (sometimes referred to as "contemporary" Munchausen syndrome by proxy): the usual motive for the mother is to prevent the father having access to the child.

Hysteria by proxy—The mother who believes herself to have an unusual allergy or incapacitating postviral syndrome and imposes the same symptoms on her child.

Delusional disorder—Mothers who have genuine mental illness and are deluded about their child's incapacity or illness.

* For further details of identification of samples by DNA markers contact: DNA Laboratory, St James's University Hospital, Leeds LS9 7TF. Tel: 0113 283 7073, Fax: 0113 246 7090.

Further reading

Meadow SR. Munchausen syndrome by proxy. *J Clin Forensic Med* 1994;**1**:121–7.
Rosenberg DA. Web of deceit: a literature review of Munchausen syndrome by proxy. *Child Abuse Negl* 1987;**11**:547–63.
Bools C, Neale B, Meadow R. A follow-up of victims of fabricated illness (Munchausen syndrome by proxy). *Arch Dis Child* 1993;**69**:625–30.
McClure RJ, Davis PM, Meadow SR, *et al*. Epidemiology of Munchausen syndrome by proxy, non-accidental poisoning and non-accidental suffocation. *Arch Dis Child* 1996;**75**:57–61.
Levin AV, Sheridan MS. *Munchausen syndrome by proxy*. New York: Lexington Books, 1995.

DILEMMAS

Roy Meadow

Child abuse runs counter to the views that most of us have of family life, the reciprocity of love between parent and child, and our belief that children fare best in their own homes with their own parents. We wish that child abuse did not happen, therefore diagnosing and reporting child abuse is a distasteful task. Even for paediatricians and child psychiatrists whose priority is the child it can be difficult; it is the more difficult for general practitioners, psychiatrists, and other specialists whose patient is the perpetrator and who may feel they are breaching confidences. Diagnosing or reporting abuse disrupts the usual trusting relationship that exists between the child's parent and the doctor, and for the medical practitioner who suggests the possibility of abuse there may follow abuse and aggravation from the family, considerable disruption to a planned work schedule because of attendance at case discussions, case conferences, and courts; as well as a lot of extra paperwork—writing reports. Therefore for most doctors there will be a tendency to underdiagnose and to underreport abuse rather than the reverse.

Confidentiality

While one understands the problems of psychiatrists and general practitioners, who have a responsibility for adult family members, of whether to inform statutory agencies about abuse and how much information to divulge at multiagency child protection case conferences, the professional and legal position is clear. The advice on medical confidentiality from the General Medical Council, the British Medical Association, and the Academy of Medical Royal Colleges is that the needs of the child must take priority.

Threshold for reporting

Though it is easy to state that *any* child abuse should be reported, experienced professionals think carefully before so doing. They worry that their suspicion of abuse may be unfounded and that investigation of their suspicion may be counterproductive and not in the child's best interests. The worries about reporting at too low a threshold are understandable because of awareness of the great upset that investigation of suspected child abuse may cause for the family. (Three quarters of parental partnerships break up within a year of an allegation of abuse.) They may also have doubts about the efficacy of the child protection procedures, which can be criticised for putting great resource into the investigation of an allegation at the expense of insufficient help for a family in difficulty. Doctors may have had experience of previous inconclusive investigations which have caused much upset. They are likely also to have seen the practical difficulty of helping children whose protection is at issue, who invariably have multiple needs, many of which cannot be met. (One third come from lone parent families; near half live in a home that lacks a wage earner; domestic violence and mental illness are common in the home.) They may also have doubts about the ability of the agencies to protect children and of the benefit of alternative parenting should that be necessary.

There are some answers to these doubts and cogent counterarguments. In relation to protection of the child the agencies have quite a good record. Moreover, while a family may have multiple problems, not all of which can be solved, it is a truism to state that if one can solve just one of a family's many problems the total of their despair may be halved.

The publicity given to children removed needlessly from their own homes is misleading in that in 96% of cases children stay at home and, even in that minority in which they are removed from parental care, over two thirds are returned to their home within the next six months. Substitute care *is* open to criticism. About 5% of children in care are eventually adopted, and, though placement of infants for adoption has an excellent outcome, it is much more problematical for older children. In relation to fostering, infants fare well and children and older teenagers do reasonably well but for those in middle childhood, about the ages of 10 or 12, there is a 50% chance of the fostering relationship breaking down. That sort of knowledge, plus the publicity given to child abuse taking place in substitute care, gives those reluctant to notify abuse an extra excuse for their inaction.

To state, as some doctors do, that to make a false positive diagnosis of child abuse is the biggest crime of all is facile. All doctors make errors in their diagnoses, and if one never made a false positive diagnosis of a common condition one would certainly be failing on many occasions to diagnose it. Secondly, it is necessary to separate the diagnostic process from the subsequent management. Consideration of abuse as a possible reason for a child's condition and including it in the list of differential diagnoses is a necessary part of everyday practice and does not constitute a false positive diagnosis. It would be a negligent doctor who never included child abuse as a possibility for many childhood presentations. Including abuse in the list of possibilities should lead to appropriate investigation—it is simple to check the child protection register, it is simple for the hospital doctor to telephone the health visitor and general practitioner, it is simple to meet other relatives, and, in the best units, it is also simple to discuss with an experienced social worker. We should be aiming for circumstances in which it is as easy for the doctor, and as acceptable for the parents, to arrange for a social work assessment as it is to arrange for the child to have computed tomography or be referred to an ear, nose, and throat specialist.

The priority is to act in the child's best interests, and, although individual doctors may have varying thresholds for diagnosis and notification, early collaboration with social services is likely to achieve a more uniform approach countrywide that serves children and their parents best. Such early collaboration is more likely when social services adopt a careful and sensitive approach to their investigation, avoiding hasty decisions or intemperate separation of childen from their parents.

Who should examine the child

A doctor may be reluctant to be involved in child abuse and slow to take on the responsibility of examining a child suspected of abuse for many reasons. Most of them are linked to either lack of training or lack of appropriate support and multidisciplinary help. A common fear of an inexperienced doctor is that he or she may jeopardise, by their interview and examination, a subsequent investigation that may be required by social services or the police.

Doctors should be reassured about their role and have clear priorities. Their chief duty is to the child and to the child's immediate wellbeing. Thus, if the child is in danger, is in pain, or requires resuscitation or special investigation get on with it, just as is the case with any other child in trouble. Appropriate medical investigation and treament must take priority over everything else. Further assessment and forensic tests are a secondary consideration, important but less important than the child's immediate safety and wellbeing. Most doctors will have access to local guidelines about what to do if they suspect or diagnose abuse. These should be followed. In the United Kingdom there will be consultant paediatricians on call who are experienced in child abuse work, and there should be a duty social worker available.

Most child abuse, however, is not an emergency and, in those circumstances, it is important to proceed cautiously and to ensure that examinations and assessments are performed in the best way. Then it is helpful to consider the check list (below) which has been provided by the Royal College of Paediatrics and Child Health Standing Committee on Child Protection.

Organised abuse

The term is used when child abuse involves a number of abusers or a number of children or both, who may incur similar or different forms of abuse. An element of organisation is involved. Thus, groups involved with distribution of child pornography (often for financial profit) and groups of adults (often incorporating family networks) who establish paedophile rings to use children for sexual gratification are examples of organised abuse.

Sometimes the organised abuse is said to be "*ritual abuse*", which means that it is linked to group activities with either religious, magical, or supernatural connotation, which is repeated and used to intimidate and coerce children. "*Satanic abuse*" is alleged when the ritual is linked to belief in and worship of Satan. Both the last two terms tend to cause confusion, and it is probably better to describe the circumstances and extent of any organised abuse rather than to use sensational terminology.

Sensational stories are popular with newspapers and have led to extravagant publicity for ritual abuse. Careful investigation usually reveals that the stories are ill founded and much exaggerated. The dilemma for investigators is that experience shows that, just because the circumstances of a child's abuse may seem too extraordinary or horrific to believe, it does not mean it has not happened. Much child abuse and the circumstances in which it is perpetrated are beyond the knowledge and imagination of normal people. It is prudent when investigating extraordinary allegations, however, to raise the threshold for diagnosis and confirmation of abuse. The more incredible the abuse the more sure one must be of the facts.

Check list to consider before examining child when abuse suspected

- Am I the right person to examine the child?
- Are there forensic implications?
- What other doctors/facilities need to be alerted to advise/support?
- Do I know how to contact them?
- Is all relevant health information available?
- Is the issue of consent clarified?
- Has the issue of confidentiality been dealt with?
- Is this the best time for the *child* to undergo the examination?
- Is the environment appropriate—is it child friendly, is privacy ensured?
- Are the right people available to support the child?

False allegations

A large proportion of allegations of abuse, particularly sexual abuse, which are investigated do not lead to further proceedings and prove to be unsubstantiated. Some are unsubstantiated because there is insufficient evidence for further action. But in other cases there is a likelihood that the allegations are false.

False allegations of abuse, particularly sexual abuse, are common at the time of parental separation and disputes concerning custody of, or access to, children. In the United States it is reported that at least one third of the allegations of abuse that are made in the context of custody disputes are false. An additional large proportion are or access to children. In the United States it is reported that at least one third of the allegations of abuse that are made in the context of custody disputes are false. An additional large proportion are unsubstantiated. The usual circumstance is the child's mother alleging sexual abuse by the father. The context is difficult because it is likely there is an increase of sexual abuse in these families, which in some cases has been the reason for separation, or in which separation has provided the circumstances in which the child may be abused. Moreover, children who did not disclose abuse before their parents separated may feel able to do so when living away from the perpetrator. Nevertheless, amid the unhappiness, bitterness, and selfishness that is evident when parents separate, false allegations are relatively common and mothers may use an allegation of abuse as a way of preventing the father having access to his children. During the protracted investigation of such cases it is common for young children to be denied access to one of their parents, usually the father, for many months or even years; and the child does then incur abuse—severe emotional abuse.

Much less common is the parent, usually the mother, who reports abuse as a way of gaining attention for herself, and for the contact which she cherishes with the child protection agencies, doctors, or police. Seemingly she is able to disregard the turmoil of investigations and assessments her false story causes for the child.

Unfounded allegations may come from relatives, neighbours, teachers, and other professionals, but usually they will have been made in a well meaning rather than in a mischievous way.

Some children give false stories of being abused. The time when a child's testimony was regarded as the absolute truth is past, and it is acknowledged that young children are vulnerable to suggestion and will elaborate on misunderstood stories originating from adults and that school children will repeat stories that they have learnt from videos. Older children and adolescents may produce an overdetailed story with extravagant, horrific, or erotic detail. For all witnesses recollection of events is altered by the passage of time, by misunderstandings, outside pressure, and sometimes intent, resulting in allegations that are untrue. Therefore, there is always more doubt about allegations that are made long after the event, those that lack intimate details and vivid experience or feeling, those without corroborative evidence, and those occurring within the context of parental disputes about custody or contact. The assessment of such testimony requires an experienced and skilled person who has a non-judgmental and open mind in relation to the accusation and the skill to elicit reliable information without reinforcing false elements by repeated questions or suggestions.

Further reading

Department of Health. *Medical responsibilities*. London: Department of Health, 1994.
Department of Health. *Child protection: messages from research*. London: HMSO, 1995.
Heiman ML. Putting the puzzle together: validating allegations of child sexual abuse. *J Child Psychol Psychiatry* 1992;**33**:311–29.
NSPCC. *Listening to children*. London: Longmans, 1990.
Meadow R. False allegations of abuse and Munchausen syndrome by proxy. *Arch Dis Child* 1993;**68**:444–7.
Papers on ritual abuse. *Child Abuse Neglect* 1992;**15**:163–96.

ROLE OF THE CHILD PSYCHIATRY TEAM

Ingrid Davison, Rory Nicol

Child psychiatrists' training in adult mental health and often, nowadays, in paediatrics as well as their experience of the development and emotional, behavioural, and social functioning of children places them in a unique position in medicine. They work in different settings across the country, but most work within a multidisciplinary team, which may include a clinical psychologist, educational psychologist, social worker, community psychiatric nurse, occupational therapist, specialist teacher, and non-medical child psychotherapist, as well as a consultant child psychiatrist. Such a child psychiatry team, working alongside and in close communication with agencies central to the investigation and management of child abuse, such as social services departments and the police, is well placed to assist in a holistic assessment of a child and its family and to offer treatment accordingly.

Why should child psychiatrists become involved in child abuse?

All forms of child abuse will have a psychological impact on the child and may affect his or her emotional, social, and behavioural adjustment and development, and are therefore of interest to the child psychiatrist. Such effects may be short term or long term but are not inevitable. Well timed treatment will modify the later outcome of

child abuse, but child psychiatrists are also aware of the importance of resilience factors in a child's life which can protect him or her against the full impact of adverse experiences. It is important to identify positive features in a child's experience as well as negative ones in the prediction of future outcome.

The box below simplifies some of the adverse emotional and behavioural effects associated with child abuse, together with possible potential outcomes in later childhood and adult life.

When should the child psychiatrist become involved in cases of child abuse?

There are several points in the management of child abuse when involvement of the child psychiatry team should be considered. A child psychiatrist is particularly likely to be helpful when he or she has extensive experience of this difficult work.

Investigation

The roles of identification and investigation of child abuse are primarily those of the social services departments and the police. It is often helpful, however, for the child psychiatry team to become involved early—for example, in more complex cases where the skill of the child psychiatrist will be of help in understanding the relationship of behaviour, emotions, and family problems to potential abuse.

Assessment

Not all cases of proven child abuse require assessment by the child psychiatric team. If the child is coping well at home and at school and has a supportive relationship with a caring adult, further intervention might be counterproductive.

An assessment by a child psychiatrist is indicated if the children in the family are presenting with emotional, behavioural, or social difficulties or a delay in development. The child psychiatrist's training and experience is such that he or she is well equipped to assess in addition parental mental health, the nature of family relationships, and, most importantly, the quality of parenting provided to the children.

In cases where there is doubt about child abuse the child psychiatrist should still be involved if there is concern about the emotional, social, and behavioural adjustment

Childhood experience	Possible outcome
Understimulation	Developmental delays
Emotional neglect	Indiscriminate overfriendliness, overactivity, and aggression Problems in making and sustaining intimate personal relationships
Emotional abuse	Disturbed feeding behaviour, wetting, and soiling Poor social adjustment Antisocial behaviour
Excessive punitiveness	Passive "frozen" behaviour Disorganised aggression
Family violence	Conduct disorder
Sexual abuse	Sexualised behaviour Self mutilation Eating disorders Depression Sexual dysfunction

and development of the child. He or she may be able to shed useful light on the probability of child abuse having occurred, which can then be investigated further by the appropriate agencies. This is particularly so when emotional abuse is suspected. Emotional abuse is defined as "the severe adverse effect on the behaviour and emotional development of a child caused by persistent or severe emotional ill treatment or rejection". Its diagnosis therefore falls squarely within the clinical remit of the child psychiatrist, who should be able to provide valuable insights into the nature and effect of such abuse.

Court work

The Children Act 1989 has placed a new emphasis on the multidisciplinary assessment of children and their families and has placed an obligation on health authorities to cooperate with social services departments in such assessments. This has led to increased demand by the courts on child psychiatrists to assess and formulate problems of child abuse within families and to advise on future management and treatment. All child psychiatrists should have skill in the presentation of complex problems in a way that can be understood by the court.

In cases which have led to a criminal prosecution, children may be expected to give evidence in court as witnesses. Use of a screen or video link may offer some protection to children facing this experience, but the adversarial nature of our legal processes takes little account of the psychological needs of children, who sometimes find their account of their abuse challenged and discredited by the very system they believed would protect them. This can be as psychologically damaging as the abuse itself. In addition, those offering therapy to a child going through this process must take care that their work cannot be misinterpreted as "coaching" the child and so "influencing the evidence".

Management

Information is needed in a variety of areas if correct decisions are to be made. These include information about the nature, severity, and effect of the abuse; the risk of continuing abuse; the quality of parenting; the quality of family relationships; and the family's potential for change. The balance between the risks of continuing abuse if the child remains with its family and the inevitable damage resulting from removal from the family must be assessed. Long term plans about child care must be made as quickly as possible and must ensure that the best interests of the child are paramount. In practice, this often means deciding which is the least damaging of several alternatives.

The training and experience of a child psychiatrist familiar with such cases can be invaluable in this decision making process. Child psychiatrists should play a part in case conferences and meetings, planning the long term management of cases in which they have become involved. This role has received new emphasis in judgments given in recent well publicised child sexual abuse cases.

In addition to collaborating in the long term management of child abuse cases, the child psychiatrist is in a good position to advise about specific treatment and management.

Treatment

It is generally accepted that the major role of the child psychiatry team in cases of child abuse is in the provision of treatment. The focus of treatment must be the welfare of the child and the improvement of parent-child relationships, even if the child is not the identified patient in treatment. These concepts may be unfamiliar to professionals who do not work regularly with abused children. Since treatment programmes are often individually tailored, it is impossible to describe all possible approaches. However, the following are particularly relevant to child abuse.

• Occasionally parental mental illness contributes to the abuse of a child. While the child psychiatrist, with training in adult mental health as well as experience of child abuse and family functioning, is in a good position to diagnose such illness, it is advisable to involve the general adult psychiatric services in treatment. The adult psychiatrist should then also be involved in planning long term management of the case, since he or she will be able to advise about the likely outcome of treatment and have access to other resources, which may be helpful.

• More commonly it is not possible to diagnose a specific mental illness, but one or both parents may show evidence of a personality disorder associated with poor quality of parenting, and inadequate control of impulses. Psychological intervention aimed at enabling parents to assume responsibility for their behaviour and to control their impulses may be helpful. A number of different professionals might take on this work, but it is often helpful to involve the local forensic psychiatry service, who are especially experienced in this area.

• Assessment of abusive families often reveals a multigenerational cycle of abuse, with parents who have experienced abuse in their own childhoods then going on to repeat similar abuse with their own children. Often parents have spoken to no one about these experiences and, once having broached the issue, are keen to have help for themselves. In such situations a referral to the local adult psychotherapy or counselling service may be helpful. Alternatively it may be necessary for the professionals working with the family, including the child psychiatric team, to address these issues with the parents before they are able to move on and improve their parenting skills. The social workers who work with the child psychiatric team often have skills and expertise particularly relevant in this area.

• Improving parenting skills is clearly an important aim when working with abusive families and can be tackled in a variety of different ways. Parents often need advice about behavioural management techniques. In abusing families the importance of praise and rewards for appropriate behaviour often needs particular emphasis, as well as the use of non-abusive sanctions for undesirable behaviour. Some child psychiatric teams have day or inpatient resources where families are admitted for observation and modification of parenting skills on a here and now basis and the clinical psychologist in the team can be particularly helpful in devising appropriate programmes. In many areas such work is undertaken in family centres run by the local social services department. The child psychiatric team can offer support and consultation to such establishments.

• Abused children often present with serious and persistent emotional and behavioural problems which require treatment if future development is to proceed. In younger children play therapy is a valuable approach, allowing the child the opportunity to explore his or her feelings about the abuse through the medium of play. In older children individual psychotherapy is treatment based on talking, which addresses the same issues, although with all children drawing and play materials can add to the therapeutic process.

• Psychotherapy is hard work that requires motivation and inner strength on the part of the child. For some children it is not an appropriate treatment, particularly for those who have been severely damaged by their experiences or those whose future remains uncertain. For these children the child psychiatric team can still offer help by working with their carers, to enable them to offer understanding and support to the children in their daily lives.

• Sexually abused children may present with sexualised behaviour which leaves them vulnerable to further abuse. It is important to undertake work with these children that will enable them to protect themselves in the future. This work usually focuses on the child's rights over his or her own body, the difference between caring and abusive touching, good and bad secrets, and strategies that the child can use to escape from potentially abusive situations. These issues are often most successfully addressed among a group of developmentally similar children, but if a group is not available there is no reason why the work cannot be undertaken on an individual basis.

• Group approaches can be helpful in the treatment of child abuse. Protective groups for sexually abused children have already been mentioned, but parent training groups, play groups for abused children, groups for mothers of sexually abused children, and groups for perpetrators are all receiving increasing attention.

• Conjoint family approaches—that is, those in which the whole family is seen together—can be useful in physical, emotional, and sexual abuse but need to be used with caution and when the aim of the treatment is clear. Their indiscriminate use by inexperienced therapists is naive and potentially damaging.

• Abuse carried out by children is receiving more recognition and is an important issue for child psychiatrists. Such children have often been abused themselves and have then gone on to abuse others. They must be helped to acknowledge responsibility for their own abusive actions and to begin to make reparation before they can then go on to explore their experiences of abuse. These children raise questions about accepted stereotypes of sexual abuse and are particularly challenging to work with.

These specific interventions should be subordinate to the overall treatment and management programme for the children and families. The process and results of treatment need to be carefully documented because, apart from the specific benefits of the treatment, they may contribute valuable information about the capacity and motivation of the family to change and hence contribute to the major multidisciplinary decisions that need to be made about the family at case conferences.

Consultation and education

Child abuse is a harrowing and disturbing aspect of modern life and not all professionals who come into contact with such cases have the training or experience to prepare them adequately. The child psychiatry team can be a useful local resource offering consultation and education to professionals in the specialty, either by means of formalised training programmes or consultation arrangements—for example, with residential children's homes or on an ad hoc case by case basis.

Further reading

Black D, Wolkind S, Hendriks JH, eds. *Child psychiatry and the law*. London: Royal College of Psychiatrists, 1989.
Furniss T. *The multiprofessional handbook of child sexual abuse*. London: Routledge, 1991.
Jones D. *Interviewing children who have been sexually abused*. 4th ed. London: Royal College of Psychiatrists, Gaskell Press, 1992.
Royal College of Psychiatrists. *The evidence of children*. London: Royal College of Psychiatrists, 1996. (Council Report No 44.)

SOCIAL WORKERS AND CHILD PROTECTION

Michael Preston-Shoot

Local authority social services departments have four major child protection duties arising from the Children Act 1989: to prevent children suffering ill treatment and neglect; to safeguard and promote the welfare of children in need; to investigate a child's circumstances when requested by a court; and (along with the National Society for the Prevention of Cruelty to Children (NSPCC)) to investigate information that a child is suffering or is likely to suffer significant harm and decide whether any action should be taken to safeguard and promote the child's welfare. Each local authority has its own procedures but must work within a general framework and the definitions of significant harm, children in need, and health and development provided in the act and elaborated in central government guidance, such as local authority circulars, much of which for social services departments has the full force of legislation. Social services departments therefore have a central role in the prevention, investigation, and management of cases of child abuse.

Local authorities vary in their organisational structures. Sometimes community based social workers are allocated referred work on the basis of geographical area served or specialism (such as short term or long term work; children and families or adult services). Sometimes practitioners are divided by role—those purchasing services and therefore involved in assessment; those providing services, packages of care agreed as part of protection plans or responses to children in need. Some local authorities also maintain hospital social work departments, where practitioners work with nominated wards, medical specialties, or consultants. Local authorities vary in the extent to which, after referral and initial investigation, hospital social workers are involved in child protection cases.

In all work with children and families the child's welfare is paramount and is determined by consideration of a welfare checklist (section 1(3) of the Children Act 1989). Social work practice operates within this framework, which seeks to balance parental responsibility and rights with children's rights and the duty of the state to intervene in certain circumstances. Five principles inform such practice.

Primacy of family—This entails promoting the upbringing of children in need by their families when consistent with the duty to safeguard and promote the child's welfare. Services may be provided to assist families—for instance, day care, family centres, and counselling. Courts will make orders only when satisfied that so doing would be better than making no order at all. Parents retain parental responsibility when a child is in care; the local authority is able to limit this only when necessary to safeguard and promote the child's welfare. Where practicable and appropriate children looked after by the local authority should be placed near home or within the extended family, or both.

Partnership—This is the most effective means of providing care for children, whatever the legal position. It means the full involvement of parents and children in assessment, decision making, and reviews. A key feature is the negotiation of written agreements which detail the purpose and content of the work to be done.

Multidisciplinary teamwork—No one

Key practice skills, emphasising partnership

- Honesty, openness, and respect

- Providing information about the purposes of interviews and available services

- Clear explanations of local authority powers and duties, reasons for concern, and what is or is not negotiable about involvement

- Clear language and preparation with families to enable their informed participation in decision making

- Engaging with the expression of strong feelings without defensiveness

- Addressing conflicts of interest directly, working with the family without compromising the child's interests

- Listening to families, entering their world, and understanding their perspective, without colluding with the family, becoming overwhelmed, or maintaining unrealistic optimism

- Planning and reviews, to avoid drift and to retain clear objectives

- Written agreements detailing the child's needs, the plan to meet these needs, the actions required by those involved, and the timescale

- Work tackles the family's concerns, values their contributions, and develops, where possible, their skills and strengths

- Recording—a detailed individual and family history cross referenced with significant events; the content and process of investigation, assessment, decision making, and intervention

- Decisions confirmed in writing

- Self awareness—monitoring the interaction between self and work, especially defence mechanisms such as avoidance of issues, defensive practice, and authoritarianism.

professional group has all the knowledge and skills required for the prevention of abuse or neglect, for child protection, or for the work required after protection. Social workers may request assistance from other professionals working with children and families, who must assist (sections 27 and 47(10), Children Act 1989) unless this is unreasonable or prejudicial to the discharge of their own functions. Area child protection committees are responsible for developing agreed objectives and procedures for interagency cooperation in case management and decision making. This is crucial since interagency dangerousness, disagreements, or conflicts between professionals undermine child protection work.

Antidiscriminatory practice—Local authority services and practice must not reflect or reinforce discrimination and must meet the special needs of particular groups (Race Relations Act 1976; Children Act 1989). Thus when decisions are made about children race, culture, religion, and linguistic background must be considered. Moreover, social workers work to counteract the impact of discrimination arising from race, sex, disability, age, poverty, and sexuality. Accordingly, work will target the impact of inequality and structural oppression on individuals and families. The power imbalance between clients and professionals will be challenged through the use of written agreements, client advocates, open records, informed participation in meetings, and attention to workers' sex, ethnicity, and use of power.

Prevention—An emphasis on abuse and child protection should not obscure other needs in a case nor the importance of providing services to children in need. Legal options should be the least coercive consistent with meeting the child's needs, including no order at all. Compulsory orders (emergency protection, child assessment, care orders) should be sought for the following reasons:

• When they are better than voluntary arrangements—that is, when services have been refused or failed, or are likely to fail, to promote the child's welfare; when there is serious risk; when assessment is frustrated
• When they are in the interests of the child—based on clearly identified needs
• After a detailed investigation and case conference which consider whether services by agreement with the family would meet the child's needs.

Emergency protection orders should not be the routine first step in response to child abuse except in situations of clear and serious risk of significant harm.

More broadly, social services departments will, through liaison with other agencies and community groups, seek to develop community networks and resources to reduce environmental pressures and promote the prevention of abuse or neglect and the protection of children.

None the less, social workers face difficult practice dilemmas. These include prevention versus protection (at what level to intervene), care versus control (how to use the law), rights versus risk (when the state should intervene), and needs versus resources (what determines decisions). Effective supervision, training, guidelines, and multidisciplinary teamwork, together with knowledge of the law and good practice, are essential for decision making in this context.

Assessment and intervention

Together with open discussion between professionals and with children and parents, minimising delay and avoiding unnecessary intervention which prejudice the child's welfare, and ongoing consideration of the child's safety, social work practice has six interlocking components.

Acquisition and collation of information through facilitative questions; observation; listening and clarification; informing decision making by placing risks to and needs of the child in the context of family history, significant events, and details of abuse or neglect. Social workers will follow the guidance given in the Cleveland report, interviewing at the child's pace, restricting the number of interviews, ensuring the suitability of the work setting, and recording carefully. Creation of a safe space (reliability, consistency, role clarity) is essential if those involved are to be enabled to provide information and to convey their feelings and experiences. Social workers will look for evidence which corroborates statements of abuse or neglect. They must avoid preconceptions and exerting undue influence on people to disclose.

Study and evaluation of information—This entails distinguishing fact from opinion and content (the "what") from process (how people have engaged with the issues), using research and theoretical knowledge, and considering the case from different perspectives. The task here

---

Risk assessment

By using agreed indicators of risk and levels of (significant) harm the objective is to determine the seriousness of risk and harm or the likelihood of risk and harm, or both. This must then be considered alongside possible interventions: balancing the effects of removing the child with the possibility of harm if not removed from home and whether a voluntary agreement with the parents is sufficient to safeguard the child's welfare.

• Low risk • Potential risk • Moderate risk	Monitoring, with clear criteria when to act; ongoing assessment; negotiated agreement sought on work to be done; legal options considered if agreement is not possible
• Cumulative risk	Legal options to protect the child considered; agreement sought on work to be done; ongoing assessment
• Acute/immediate risk	May warrant immediate removal of the child.

Assessing prospects for rehabilitation

Checklists have been developed to identify families where the rehabilitation of abused children might be indicated. No checklist is foolproof. Care must be taken that they do not oppress families by the inappropriate imposition of white eurocentric norms and the exclusion of structural issues (such as racism, poverty, unemployment, and housing). Each case must be considered alongside the availability of research knowledge. However, checklists do emphasise the factors that must be included in this type of assessment:

- What was the nature, frequency, and severity of the abuse or neglect?

- Has the abuse stopped? Is there a culture of violence or aggression in the family? How are relationships and decisions managed? How is power used?

- Do the parents accept responsibility and the need for change? Can they work for this change?

- Is there open communication about the abuse or neglect and about family problems? Are there substantial family problems? To what extent are the parents able to meet the child's needs? Is there a distinction between the child's needs and parents' needs? Are expectations of children realistic?

- Can the child resist any abuse? Has the child non-abusive supports available?

- Have the child's views been sought, worked with, and considered? Is the child fearful or requesting protection? Is the child accommodating to the abusing or neglectful parent?

- What has been the outcome of previous work with the family, if any?

is to understand and appraise the available information. For instance, what is the effect of parental behaviour on the child? What awareness is there in the family of the child's needs? What networks are available to support this family? How cooperative have the parents been with professionals?

Formulation of assessment—This entails defining and clarifying problems and weighing up risks, needs, and resources. A needs assessment focuses on the child and the family, with special reference to the child's health and development (physical and mental health and social, emotional, educational, physical, and behavioural development) and environmental stresses (housing, income, race, and social and community networks). Resource assessment includes those resources available to the family and those resources within the professional network which might enable risks to be decreased, problems resolved, and needs met. An initial investigation and assessment will consider the sources and levels of risk or harm, or both, and the grounds for concern, culminating in recommendations of how best to protect the child, including the legal options most likely to promote this. Where an investigation and assessment rule out abuse or neglect, everyone involved must be informed in writing and services offered to children in need and their families. A comprehensive assessment, when requested by a court or case conference to provide the basis for decisions

about the future management of the case, will gather and evaluate information on the areas of concern: the child's health and development; the family's resources, strengths, and problems; family interactions and the ability to meet the child's needs; and available support networks. Again, recommendations will be made about what needs to change to reduce the risk to the child or meet his or her needs, or both, and what form of intervention is most likely to achieve this.

Child protection plan—A statement about the work's objectives and how these are to be achieved. These plans should include the child's needs (including education, health, and race); how these needs are to be met; services to be provided, including placements, with their aims and timescales; arrangements for contact between child and family; arrangements for consulting the child, parents, and significant others and how they are to be involved in decision making; responsibility for implementing the plan; contingency plans if the plan or placement breaks down; and review dates.

Intervention with individuals (child, non-abusing parent, perpetrator) or families, or both. Therapeutic work may entail play therapy with children, family therapy, or the use of group work with, say, survivors or perpetrators of abuse. The objectives of intervention may be to decrease risks of abuse or neglect, to improve an individual's or family's strengths and resources, or to work through the effects of abuse or neglect. Intervention, when a child has been removed from home, may aim to test the prospects for rehabilitation or, if return home has been excluded, to work towards a permanent placement. The first six weeks are crucial in the consideration of rehabilitation or permanent placement if work is to remain focused and purposeful.

Review—This entails involving parents, children, and relevant other people involved in the case to evaluate progress achieved, to reconsider the child protection plan and whether any change is necessary in the child's legal status, and to establish the framework and content of forthcoming work to safeguard and promote the child's welfare. Written notification of the outcome must be given to those involved in the case. Reviews demonstrate that assessment is an ongoing process involving the child, family, and professional network.

Contact

The frequency and length of contact between social workers and families varies. During initial investigations it can be daily for several hours. When meetings between children looked after by the local authority and their parents are supervised it can amount to several times each week over a considerable period. Contact during assessments is often weekly, with comprehensive assessments requiring between eight and 12 weeks. Frequency and length of contact at the intervention stage will vary considerably depending on the method and focus of the work. Concerns exist that social workers are underresourced; in particular that the time involved in initial investigations, child protection assessments, recording, and court work limits resources for intervention after

assessment or work with children and families when need rather than abuse is the focus.

Further reading

Braye S, Preston-Shoot M. *Practising social work law.* 2nd ed. London: Macmillan, 1997.
Butler-Sloss E. *Report of the inquiry into child abuse in Cleveland.* London: HMSO, 1988.
Department of Health. *Child protection. Messages from research.* London: HMSO, 1995.
Department of Health. *The challenge of partnership in child protection: practice guide.* London: HMSO, 1995.
Parker R, Ward H, Jackson S, *et al.* eds. *Looking after children. Assessing outcomes in child care.* London: HMSO, 1991.

CASE CONFERENCES

Michael Preston-Shoot

Case conferences are central to assessment, interagency cooperation, and decision making in child protection. They are convened by social services departments (and sometimes the NSPCC) when an initial investigation has confirmed or suspected abuse or neglect. To be effective their decisions must follow from consideration of all the available information, including a detailed individual and family history cross referenced with significant family events and an appraisal of the family's ability to protect the child and willingness to cooperate with professionals.

Except in relation to registration and the appointment of a key worker, case conferences make recommendations to participant agencies. These agencies should follow locally agreed procedures for confirming their intention to implement these recommendations. The key worker will be a local authority or NSPCC social worker. He or she may not be the person most in contact with the family but will ensure that the child protection plan is developed and implemented and is central to interagency work: coordinating agency contributions to assessment, intervention, and review; engaging the child and parents in the child protection plan; and facilitating communication between agencies.

Confidentiality

Confidentiality is a key question since effective intervention and case management depend on consideration of all available information. Child protection inquiries commonly pinpoint the failure to disclose or ask for information as crucial in distorting assessment and decision making.

Codes of confidentiality issued by the General Medical Council, the British Association of Social Workers, and the United Kingdom Central Council for Nursing, Midwifery and Health Visiting allow disclosure and confirm the duty to share information when there is reason to believe a person is being abused or that serious danger exists. The paramount duty is the protection of the child.

Composition of case conferences

Case conferences include those with specific child protection responsibilities and those with a contribution to make to the specific case.

Chairperson—This is a senior member of the social services department (occasionally the NSPCC), with detailed knowledge and understanding of child protection and without line management responsibility for the case now or previously. When possible the same person should chair all case conferences concerning particular children and families. The chairperson ensures the conference prioritises the child's interests, clarifies the meeting's purpose and the roles of people present, and facilitates each person to contribute verbally and by reports.

NSPCC—Some staff attend as observers or consultants when not directly involved in the case. They may provide comprehensive assessments to inform decision making, or resources such as family centres and family therapy.

Social workers and team leader report on the initial investigation and provide background information; they are responsible for ensuring that everyone with a relevant contribution to make has been invited; and they collate and record all available information.

Education welfare officers are sometimes concerned directly in an investigation or able to provide information about the family, or both, especially the child's school attendance and performance.

Teachers, nursery and playgroup workers, and childminders often observe symptoms of abuse or neglect; they may be the first to whom a child discloses abuse.

Police will provide information on any suspected individual discussed at the

---

Tasks of case conferences

- To share and coordinate information and concerns about the child and family, to assess the severity of abuse and neglect, and to evaluate the degree of risk

- To fulfil statutory obligations for the protection of children

- To formulate an agreed, recommended plan of management and intervention that addresses the abuse or neglect, risks, and needs in the case, with the child's welfare and safety the paramount aim. This must include consideration of what legal action is necessary to protect the abused or neglected child and other children in the family and what services should be provided on the basis of assessed needs

- To decide whether to place the child's name on the child protection register (see p 3) and to nominate a key worker (see p 3)

- To agree if and when a child protection review is required—no more than six months from the initial case conference when the child's name has been placed on the register

Reasons for family involvement

● Parental understanding of concerns, expectations, and recommendations has positive results

● Partnership increases parents' confidence and cooperation, promotes parental responsibility, and enhances the family's commitment to the child protection plan, thereby improving the chances of child protection

● Involvement reduces conflict and improves relationships between professionals and families

● Family members can provide or correct information, resulting in more informed recommendations

conference and, when officers have been coworkers with social workers in the initial investigation, will report on their assessment after interviews with the child, parents, or other people concerned. Serious assault on or abuse or neglect of a child should be reported so that officers can investigate and consider prosecution.

General practitioner—Whether or not concerned directly in the initial investigation the general practitioner has a diagnostic role concerning injuries or a child's health and development and has significant knowledge of the child and family. This will assist the conference in appraising risk and needs.

Hospital doctors are sometimes the first to suspect or identify abuse or neglect. They will advise the conference on diagnosis and on whether the signs and symptoms observed are attributable to care given by parents or carers to the child.

Health visitors, school nurses, and nurse managers contribute knowledge of the child and family. They may contribute to the child protection plan, especially when this entails monitoring a child's health and development. The nurse manager provides support and represents this part of community health services.

Probation officers may be working with family members or able to provide information about previous or possible involvement with the family (for example, work with offenders or marital work).

Voluntary organisations may be involved when they provide or could offer services to children and families.

Armed services are involved when cases have a service connection.

The circumstances of the case may indicate the involvement of other agencies or professionals: the local authority housing department, especially when there are rent arrears, overcrowding, or questions of homelessness; the Department of Social Security, where financial difficulties are significant; clinical medical officers and doctors working in the community—for instance, in schools—who are well placed to detect signs and symptoms of abuse or neglect; psychiatrists and members of community mental handicap teams; and hospital nursing staff.

Case conferences must have available specialist advice: a lawyer from the local authority's legal section; a psychiatrist and psychologist or paediatrician, or both; and interpreters and specialists working with disabled people and people from minority ethnic groups. Their role is to contribute to informed decision making—for example, about legal options; the significance and treatment of medical symptoms and signs; and the cultural components of a case.

Once a court has granted an emergency protection or interim care order and appointed a guardian *ad litem*, this officer of the court, whose role is to advise the court on issues of case management, to represent the interests of the child, and to provide courts with an independent social work perspective, may attend as an observer.

General practitioners and hospital doctors may claim a fee for attendance at case conferences.

Parental attendance

Parents and children must be invited to attend case conferences unless the chairperson decides that their exclusion is justified—for children because of their age and understanding; for parents when attendance would preclude proper consideration of the child's interests. This includes the likelihood of the conference being disrupted, violence towards professionals or the child, or undue influence being exerted by parents on a child. It does not include the possibility of prosecution. The reasons for exclusion should be recorded in the child's file.

When the interests of parents and children conflict the child's interests have priority. If parents and children are not present the conference must receive or ask for a report of their views (a written report, statement, or audio tape) and ensure that they receive details of the discussion and recommendations.

Local child protection procedures, agreed by area child protection committees, will detail how parental and child attendance, ideally for the entire conference (although separate attendance may be necessary) should be facilitated. Including parents and children exemplifies the Children Act's commitment to partnership and requires professionals to address envisaged problems, such as sharing confidential information, through training and procedural preparations.

Meaningful family participation can be facilitated by the following:

● Partnership underpinning all work with the family—openness, consultation, and consideration of wishes and views expressed
● Leaflets explaining the nature and purpose of case conferences
● Training for professionals
● Preparatory work with children and parents on their contribution to case conferences
● Assistance to facilitate attendance—for example, timing, venue, fares, and creche facilities

- Enabling parents and children to bring an advocate to support and advise them
- Written reports from professionals which distinguish facts and observations from opinions
- Active chairing—introducing the participants, clarifying purposes, and ensuring language is "client friendly"
- Open discussion about the nature and degree of risks and the resources required, including those from the family, to implement the recommended plan
- Provision of minutes and written notification of decisions and recommendations, with follow up to clarify any outstanding issues. Minutes should contain details of the unresolved issues of child protection, the interagency work necessary to deal with these, and how the child protection plan is related to the identified needs and risks.

Child protection review

Initial case conferences agree outline protection plans. Review meetings finalise the child protection plan after a comprehensive assessment or review of the plan, making changes where necessary, by considering current risks and needs in the family and whether the plan continues to protect the child. They review interagency cooperation and consider if registration should be continued or terminated. The usual interval between these reviews will be at least six months, but anyone may request a review at any time. The same requirements concerning parental and child attendance apply here. Once the child protection plan has been agreed a core group of professionals will be identified as key, essential contributors to these reviews. The group will organise case discussions and planning meetings between reviews, the frequency determined by the complexity of the case.

Factors necessary for effective child protection meetings

- Shared values and purposes
- Theoretical agreement about child protection issues
- Cooperation based on agreed roles, acceptance and understanding of differences (work focus) and agency structures (decision making), and negotiating overlap of areas of skill
- Recognising and working with, not avoiding, conflict or difference
- Adequate preparation, consistent membership or attendance, and no key absences. Clarity of decision making responsibility
- Chairperson who focuses the meeting on the task and, when appropriate, enables the meeting to consider group dynamics issues
- Absence of jargon and professional mystique, recognition of anxiety and stress in child protection work, explicit discussion of degrees of risk when appropriate, and willingness to reappraise professional (status and power) and sex stereotypes
- Careful timing of meetings to facilitate attendance
- Adequate recording of discussion, facts, decisions, recommendations, tasks, and interagency plans

Statutory reviews

When children are being looked after by the local authority statutory reviews are required after the first four weeks, three months, and every six months thereafter. They may be combined with child protection reviews. Parents and children are invited to attend, separately when this is indicated, with an officer of the social services department (not the social worker or team leader) responsible for coordinating the review and reports, including annual health reports. The local authority is required to consult and consider the views of the child, parents, and other people relevant to the case, including health care professionals. The child's views about the attendance of professionals at these reviews must be considered. Each review must reappraise the plan for the child, including case objectives, any variations to the child's placement, legal status, contact with family, and education and health needs. A formal record is made of the review, and the results sent to those concerned in the case.

Area child protection committees

The role of area child protection committees may be described as follows:

- To determine and review arrangements for working together—developing clear policies on roles and responsibilities in prevention, assessment, investigation, and treatment of child abuse and neglect; and publishing these procedures, including the principle of including parents and children at all conferences
- To develop and review joint training—covering assessment, investigation, and treatment; issues of race and sex; children with disabilities; how feelings about abuse affect practice; and professional stereotypes
- To encourage and review interagency cooperation
- To develop and review arrangements for expert advice
- To review and when necessary inquire into cases
- To monitor case conferences and the implementation of legal procedures
- To publish an annual report.

The core membership comprises senior officers or professionals, with delegated decision making powers, from the social services department, NSPCC, police, probation service, district health authority, and nursing profession; and representatives from general practice, paediatrics, and psychiatry; family health services authority; local education authority; armed services (when appropriate); and education. Other agencies which may be involved include voluntary organisations, housing departments, the Department of Social Security, and those with particular skill, for instance in religious, ethnic, and cultural matters.

The representatives pass reports and recommendations to their own agencies, and inform the area child protection committee of their agency's work in child protection.

Further reading

Bridge Child Care Consultancy Service. *Sukina. An evaluation report of the circumstances leading to her death*. London: BCCCS, 1991.

Corby B, Mills C. Child abuse: risks and resources. *Br J Social Work* 1986;**16**:531–42.

Department of Health. *Working together under the Children Act 1989. A guide to arrangements for inter-agency co-operation for the protection of children from abuse*. London: HMSO, 1991.

Kaganas F, King M, Piper C, eds. *Legislating for harmony partnership under the Children Act 1989*. London: Jessica Kingsley, 1995.

Reder P, Duncan S, Gray M. *Beyond blame—child abuse tragedies revisited*. London: Routledge, 1993.

CHILD CARE LAW

Barbara Mitchels

Child abuse can be physical, sexual, or emotional. Just as forms of abuse vary, so do the needs of each child and the family. The Children Act 1989 (Children Act) radically reformed child care law, embodying principles of cooperation and negotiation between professionals and families in child protection, also imposing a duty on local authorities to provide a wide range of assistance and services for children in need and their families. The Act created a court comprising three tiers, the High Court, county court, and magistrates court, each with concurrent jurisdiction. Cases can move up or down the tiers as necessary. The Act was followed by subsidiary legislation, rules, case law, and Guidance, indicating how its provisions are to be implemented.

Reference material which may be of interest is listed at the end of this chapter.

Underlying principles of the Children Act

Non-intervention

The Children Act encourages negotiation and cooperation between parents, children, and professionals, enabling children to remain within their own families with an appropriate input of resources rather than removing them to alternative accommodation. The emphasis is on empowering families rather than paternalistic control. The act creates several new private and public law orders, giving the court a wide choice of possibilities with which to meet the needs of a child, but it also insists that the court shall make no order unless it is better for the child to do so than making no order at all. In each case the court has to ask itself the question "Do we need to make an order to safeguard this child's health and welfare?"

Avoidance of delay

Delay is deemed to be contrary to the interests of the child and to be avoided unless absolutely necessary. Courts control timing, using "directions hearings" in which formal agreement is reached about who are the parties, notice, filing and service of evidence and reports, and dates of future hearings. Expert witnesses need to inform the court of dates when they are available to carry out assessments and, later, to give evidence. The directions given may also cover the time available for an assessment or report, funding, instructions, disclosure of information to experts, consent issues, venue of medical or psychiatric examinations, who will accompany a child, and the person(s) to whom the results should be given.

The welfare of the child is of paramount importance

The welfare of the child is the paramount consideration for the court. The Children Act contains a checklist setting out issues to which the court must have regard in making decisions about care, supervision, contact, and certain contested private law orders. Reference to this checklist during the writing of court reports, even when it is not compulsory to do so, ensures that the report is in line with the principles of the Act and is welcomed by the court.

'Family Proceedings' Under the Children Act 1989

Matrimonal Causes Act 1973
divorce
nullity/judical separation

Adoption Act 1976
Adoption proceedings

Family Law Act 1996
Divorce, separation, domestic violence etc

Part I Children Act 1989
parental responsibility ss 2-4
guardianship s 5

MCA 1973
Ancillary matters

Human Fertilisation & Embryology Act 1990
Parental Orders

Menu of orders available in Family Proceedings

residence, contact, specific issue, & prohibited steps (s 8)

parental responsibility (s 4)

appointment of guardian (s 5)

family assistance orders (s 16)

direction to local authority to investigate child's circumstances, (s 37)

welfare report (s 7)

Children Act 1989 section numbers given in parenthesis

Family Homes & Domestic Violence Act 1995

Domestic Violence & Matrimonial Proceedings Act 1976

Matrimonial Homes Act 1983
County court & High Court injuctions

Domestic Proceedings, Magistrates' Courts Act 1978
maintainance & physical protection of partners & children

Part II Children Act 1989
S 8 Orders:-
Contact
Prohibited steps
Residence
Specific issue

Change of surname s 13
Removal from jurisdiction, s 13
Family assistance orders s 16

Part IV Children Act 1989
Care s 31
Supervision s 35
Care Contact orders s 34
Education Supervision Order, s 36

Domestic Proceedings, Magistrates' Courts Act 1978
physical matters relating to children (eg with whom they are to live)

Applications listed outside the central box are 'family proceedings' as defined by the Children Act 1989.
Orders listed in the central box are available in family proceedings.

One of our leading judges said "A child is a person, not an object of concern". Clearly, children cannot always be sufficiently objective to know what is best for them, therefore their wishes and feelings cannot form the sole basis for the court's decision, but a child's views should be ascertained and taken seriously. Even very young children can indicate feelings by non-verbal means, but skill is required in interpretation. One of the tasks of a court welfare officer or a guardian *ad litem*, assisted whenever necessary by expert evidence, is to advise the court of the child's wishes and feelings and also to make a recommendation to the court as to the action most appropriate to safeguard and promote the welfare of the child (see checklist on p 67).

Parental responsibility

The Children Act changed the legal relationship between all parents and their children. It created the concept of "parental responsibility", defined in section 3(1) as "all the rights, duties, powers, responsibilities and authority which by law the parent of a child has in relation to a child and his property". Parental responsibility is the legal basis for making decisions about a child, including consent for medical treatment. The Act's provisions do not give all parents parental responsibility for their children.

Mothers and married fathers—Every mother of a child born to her (married or not) and a father married to the child's mother at the time of their child's birth or subsequently has parental responsibility for their child, which can be shared with others, but will be lost only by death or adoption.

Unmarried fathers—Unmarried fathers, who do not automatically have parental responsibility for their child, may acquire it in one of several ways:

● By written agreement with the child's mother in a formal "Parental Responsibility Agreement" signed by both parties, witnessed by an officer at court, then registered at Somerset House. Copies may be obtained for a fee, in the same way as a birth certificate
● A court order for parental responsibiity if the mother will not sign an agreement
● Parental responsibility may be given along with a residence order directing the child to live with the father, or guardianship.

The court also has power, if necessary for the child's welfare, to remove parental responsibility given by agreement or court order.

Acquisition of parental responsibility by others—Others may acquire parental

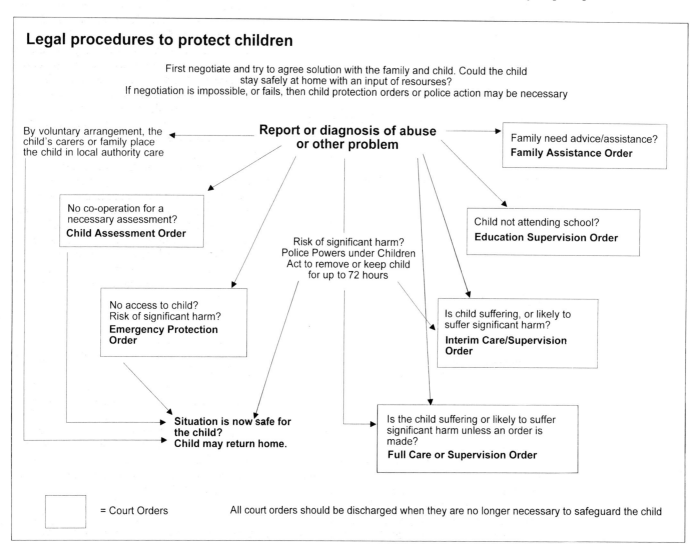

Legal procedures to protect children

First negotiate and try to agree solution with the family and child. Could the child stay safely at home with an input of resources? If negotiation is impossible, or fails, then child protection orders or police action may be necessary

Report or diagnosis of abuse or other problem

By voluntary arrangement, the child's carers or family place the child in local authority care

Family need advice/assistance?
Family Assistance Order

No co-operation for a necessary assessment?
Child Assessment Order

Child not attending school?
Education Supervision Order

Risk of significant harm? Police Powers under Children Act to remove or keep child for up to 72 hours

No access to child? Risk of significant harm?
Emergency Protection Order

Is child suffering, or likely to suffer significant harm?
Interim Care/Supervision Order

Situation is now safe for the child?
Child may return home.

Is the child suffering or likely to suffer significant harm unless an order is made?
Full Care or Supervision Order

☐ = Court Orders   All court orders should be discharged when they are no longer necessary to safeguard the child

---

Definitions of the terms used in the Children Act

Harm	Ill treatment or the impairment of health and development
Development	Physical, intellectual, social, emotional, or behavioural development
Health	Physical or mental health
Ill treatment	Includes sexual abuse and forms of ill treatment that are not physical

---

Welfare checklist (from section 1(3) Children Act 1989)

- The ascertainable wishes and feelings of the child concerned (considered in the light of his age and understanding).
- His physical, emotional, and educational needs.
- The likely effect on him of any change in his circumstances.
- His age, sex, background, and any characteristics of his which the court considers relevant.
- Any harm that he has suffered or is at risk of suffering.
- How capable each of his parents, and any other person in relation to whom the court considers the question to be relevant, is in meeting his needs.
- The range of powers available to the court under this Act in the proceedings in question.

---

responsibility along with a residence order or guardianship. A local authority may acquire parental responsibility for a child under a care order. More than one person can have parental responsibility for a child at the same time, and they will then share it.

There is an additional provision in section 3(5) of the Act that those without parental responsibility may "do what is reasonable in all the circumstances to safeguard and promote the welfare" of a child in their care, allowing a baby sitter, foster carer, or neighbour to take a child in their care for medical help in an emergency.

Medical or psychiatric examination or assessment of children

A distinction must be made at the outset between examinations and assessments for diagnosis and treatment and those purely for forensic purposes.

Examinations for diagnosis or treatment of children

In so far as general (non-emergency) treatment is concerned, consent will be required from a person having parental responsibility for a young child; and if an older child is competent to make his own medical decisions, the practitioner may also accept consent from the child. Examinations carried out without such consent could constitute an assault and could render the practitioner liable for assault in civil or criminal law, or both. When emergency treatment is required, practitioners may rely on their own clinical judgment if those in a position to give consent are unavailable. Aside from emergencies, if a practitioner considers assessment or treatment necessary and consent

is not forthcoming from any of those entitled to give it, the High Court may use its powers to act in the best interests of a child under 18 and may authorise the requisite assessment or treatment. If a problem arises for a medical practitioner concerning consent the legal department of the local authority or health service may provide legal and practical advice.

Courts control examinations for forensic purposes

Repeated medical and psychiatric examinations for forensic purposes can cause a child further unnecessary stress. The Children Act empowers the court in the context of proceedings for emergency protection, child assessment, interim care, and supervision to regulate such examinations and make appropriate directions, which may include nomination of the practitioner(s) to carry out the examination or assessment, the venue, those to be present, and those to whom the results may be given. Any unauthorised evidence obtained without observing this rule may be disallowed in court.

Child's right to refuse examinations and assessments

A child may make an informed decision to refuse an examination or assessment even if it has been authorised by the court. A child's ability to refuse will depend on factors including age, understanding, and also on the the information given. Practitioners should ensure that a child competent to make a decision is given an explanation appropriate for their age of what is proposed and the potential consequences of refusal. A note should be made of the information given to the child and of the substance of the questions and answers on which the practitioner's assessment of the child's capability to make decisions is based. That note may be later required in court if the child's capability is questioned. In care, supervision, child assessment, or emergency protection proceedings a guardian *ad litem* will have been appointed at an early stage, and will assist the court in ascertaining the child's views. When a child is brought to the doctor in accordance with a direction of the court, but then refuses, the examination should not proceed, but the matter should be referred back to the court.

Emergency protection order

Anyone may obtain this order if the court is satisfied that there is reasonable cause to believe that a child is likely to suffer significant harm unless he or she is removed from the present accommodation or if not kept at the present accommodation. This could meet the need to remove a child from home or to keep a child in hospital. Local authorities have an additional ground if they cannot gain access in respect of a child who might be suffering significant harm. The order lasts eight days initially, with the possibility of a further extension of seven days only. Anyone may apply for this order, including, therefore, a medical practitioner, but usually it will be the local authority or the police. It may be granted without notice and by a single justice. There is no appeal but after 72 hours it may be challenged in specified circumstances.

On application for an emergency protection order the court appoints a guardian *ad litem* for the child, giving directions as necessary for entry and search, disclosure of the child's whereabouts, medical examinations, and contact. Police or medical practitioners may be asked to help in carrying out the order. The applicant gains limited parental responsibility for the child, who may be looked after in local authority accommodation or hospital. The child must be returned home as soon as it becomes safe to do so. If necessary, renewal or another protective order must be sought before the order expires.

Police power to remove a child to a safe place or to prevent a child's removal from a safe place

Police have power under the Children Act to remove a child to suitable accommodation for 72 hours when there is reasonable cause to believe that the child would otherwise be likely to suffer significant harm. The police may intervene to ensure that a child in need of care is taken from home to hospital or another safe place; or to prevent the removal of a child when someone with parental responsibility is attempting to remove the child from hospital. The 72 hour duration allows time for further investigation of the child's circumstances and for a court order to be sought where necessary.

Care and supervision

There is now only one way for a child to be taken into statutory care—the court must be satisfied of the grounds laid down in section 31 of the Children Act and an order must be necessary to safeguard the child. Care orders are no longer an option in matrimonial or criminal proceedings. A care order may last until a child reaches 18 or discharged earlier on application to the court. Supervision orders may last for one year, with possible extensions for up to one year at a time, to a maximum of three years.

The grounds for care and supervision are the same, and only a local authority or authorised person (currently NSPCC) may apply. The court must have regard to the welfare checklist, the principles of non-intervention and avoidance of delay, and be satisfied that:

● The child concerned is suffering or likely to suffer significant harm
● That the harm, or likelihood of harm, is attributable to (i) the care being given or likely to be given, if an order were not made, not being what it would be reasonable to expect a parent to give; or (ii) the child being beyond parental control.

The threshold criteria for care and supervision are measured objectively against a reasonable standard of parenting. Not only must the existence or likelihood of significant harm be found, but this must be attributable to the standard of parenting experienced by the child falling below acceptable levels or the child being beyond parental control. The question of whether harm which depends on health or development is of sufficient degree to be "significant" is measured by comparison with "that which could reasonably be expected of a similar child."

Interim care/supervision orders

Interim orders may last for an initial period of up to eight weeks, followed by extensions of up to four weeks at a time. The court is anxious to avoid delay and will be unhappy about continued extensions without very good reason. Directions about contact with family and carers and medical or psychiatric assessment may be given on the making of an interim order.

Directions for medical and psychiatric examination and assessment

The court has power to order, control, or to forbid medical and psychiatric examinations and assessments when making interim orders. The directions can cover who is to carry out the assessment, venue, those accompanying the child, and disclosure of results. As discussed earlier in emergency protection orders, the child may make an informed decision to refuse, in which case the advice and help of the guardian *ad litem* should be sought and the matter should be referred back to the court.

Child assessment orders

Section 43 of the Children Act creates the child assessment order, intended for situations when a local authority has access to a child but there is a lack of cooperation from the child's carers in allowing an assessment to take place. If the child is thought to be at risk of significant harm but in no immediate danger requiring removal or retention in a safe place (for example, a long term, ongoing situation requiring further assessment) then this order may assist. As for care and supervision only the local authority or an authorised person may apply. Notice must be given to allow parties to make arrangements to attend. The court would have to be satisfied of the risk to the child and the need for the order and to be informed of previous unproductive attempts to negotiate with the family. The order may last up to seven days, during which the child may go away from home but this should be only when absolutely necessary for the assessment to take place. On hearing an application for a child assessment order the court may decide instead to make an emergency protection order if the circumstances warrant it.

Private law orders

The chart on p 65 shows proceedings designated by section 8(3)–(4) of the Act as "family proceedings" within which the court has power to make the wide range of orders indicated. Some of these, colloquially referred to as "section 8 orders" (residence, contact, specific issue, and prohibited steps) and family assistance orders may be made by the court of its own volition. In private law applications, when the issues are between individuals rather than public law when the state intervenes in a family's life, there are certain restrictions on those who may seek an order. Some are entitled to apply, some need leave. There is insufficient space to deal with this in detail here, but in most cases, with the leave of the court, anyone may apply for the section 8 orders listed above. Special restrictions apply to local authority foster parents.

Care, supervision, and emergency protection are included within "family proceedings". In the course of these cases the court has to consider all its options, therefore any expert witness needs to have them in mind too. The court will first consider whether it needs to make an order at all and then which would be the best for the child. Any description of private law orders here must necessarily be limited to a brief indication of their effects.

Residence

"An order settling the arrangements to be made as to the person with whom a child is to live", section 8. The order attaches to a person not a place. Residence may be shared—for example, to the mother during term time and to the father in the school holidays. Parental responsibility may be granted, with a residence order, to those who do not otherwise have it, and this will subsist along with the order. There are special provisions for natural fathers. Anyone with a residence order in their favour may take the child out of the country for up to one month for holiday purposes. Otherwise when there is a residence order, removal of the child from the country or a change of surname will require the written consent of all those with parental responsibility or leave of the court.

Contact

"An order requiring the person with whom a child lives or is to live, to allow the child to visit or stay with the person named in the order, or for the child and that person to have contact with each other", section 8. Contact includes telephone calls, tape and video recordings, letters, parcels, and any other form of communication.

There is a different contact order available under section 34 to regulate contact with a child in statutory care. This has special provisions of its own.

Specific issue

"An order giving directions for the purpose of determining a question which has arisen, or which may arise, in connection with any aspect of parental responsibility for a child", section 8. This order is designed to resolve disputes between those with decision making power in a child's life, who cannot resolve their disagreements by negotiation. A local authority, or anyone with leave of the court, may use this provision to seek a ruling from the court on issues such as medical treatment. Application for specific issue to the High Court could be used when those with parental responsibility for a young child refuse to allow a medical treatment which medical experts consider necessary in the interests of the child. A local authority may seek a specific issue or prohibited steps order in the best interests of a child, including a child voluntarily accommodated by them, but not in respect of a child who is subject to a care order. A local authority cannot use these orders to get care, supervision, or parental responsibility for a child.

Prohibited steps

"An order that no step which could be taken by a parent in meeting his parental responsibility for a child, and which is of a kind specified by the order, shall be taken by any person without the consent of the court", section 8. This order operates rather like an injunction and is useful, for example, when a parent is threatening to take a child out of the country without consent. It may be obtained in emergencies without notice.

Child protection referrals

Practitioners who suspect abuse, or are concerned about the health or safety of a child, should refer the child/family to the social services duty officer either in the area in which the child resides or in the hospital or to the local authority legal department. Referrals should be confirmed in writing within 24 hours. In emergencies, the police child protection unit may be notified and requested to use their powers under the Children Act. Local Area Child Protection Committee guidelines set out the basis for interdisciplinary cooperation and agreed local child protection procedures, and *Working Together* (see below) provides authoritative guidance on procedure, including child protection conferences. If practitioners are asked to give information for a child protection conference, a report should be provided, particularly if they are unable to attend. Advice may be sought from the legal department of the local authority.

Further reading

Department of Health. *An introductory guide for the NHS to the Children Act 1989.* London: Department of Health, 1989.
Home Office, Department of Health, Department of Education and Science, Welsh Office. *Working together under the Children Act 1989.* London: HMSO, 1991.
Mitchels B, Prince A. *The Children Act 1989 and medical practice.* Jordans Family Law, 1992.
NHS Management Executive. *Consent to examination and treatment.* London: Department of Health, 1990.
The care of children; principles and practice in regulations and guidance. London: HMSO, 1989.
The Children Act 1989 guidance and regulations. Vol 1. *Court orders.* London: HMSO, 1991.
The Children Act 1989 guidance and regulations. Vol 6. *Children with disabilities.* London: HMSO, 1991.

MEDICAL REPORTS

Roy Meadow, Barbara Mitchels

Notification

A doctor who is worried that a child has been abused should telephone the head of the local social work department, whether the department is in the hospital, is a community district department, or is in the legal department of the local authority. If the case is urgent action may be required immediately. Always immediately follow up the conversation with a brief letter stating the cause of concern so that there is no chance of it being forgotten. The letter, marked confidential, may be brief but should be written in language understandable to a non-medical person.

Medical reports

Formal reports are required by the courts whenever medical evidence is being used in child abuse cases. Great care must be taken over the construction of the report so that fact and opinion are clear. Sometimes a solicitor will ask you to address particular issues in detail, but quite often the doctor is asked merely for a "medical report".

Format

The report should be typed in double spacing with wide margins. It is useful to number the paragraphs or sections consecutively so that they can be referred to easily during discussion or in court.

Children Act statements

The document should be headed

In the . . . . . . court
Case Ref No . . . . . .
Re . . . (name of child, date of birth, age).
In the top right hand corner put
Filed on behalf of . . . .
Statement No . . . .
Date . . . .

And at the end the following:

"I . . . (full name) . . . declare that the content of this statement is true to the best of my knowledge, information and belief, and I understand that it may be placed before the court".

Affidavits

An affidavit is a statement of evidence set out in a standard format that has evolved over many years and is approved by the courts. It has to be sworn, or declared, before a commissioner for oaths or other authorised officer (which includes all solicitors and some court officers); a small fee is payable.

Documents or copies of documents that are relevant to the case may become part of an affidavit as exhibits, and copies may be made for all the parties to the case and for the judge. If an expert is asked to prepare a report for a civil case the report (if it is to be used in evidence) will be put into the form of an affidavit by the solicitor for the party calling the expert witness and disclosed to the other side. The evidence may then be agreed, in which case the witness need not attend the trial and the affidavit can be read. Alternatively the evidence may not be agreed and the witness may be called to court to give oral evidence. Oral evidence of expert witnesses may then be limited to the reports that have been disclosed but not agreed, saving the court's time.

Affidavits are not required in Children Act cases but are still used in other civil actions in the county court and High Court.

Criminal cases

Reports for criminal proceedings have their own format, on the requirements of which the Crown Prosecution Service will advise.

Report checklist

Name

Practising address

Work Tel No/Fax No

Professional position or appointments held

Qualifications

Relevant experience

Confidentiality checked—authority for child's address to be disclosed?

Welfare checklist—does the report take this into account?

List of people interviewed or consulted in connection with the preparation of this report with appropriate details: times, dates, location, frequency, when relevant

List of places visited in the preparation of the report, with details when relevant

List of samples taken for the preparation of the report, with details if relevant of the times and places the samples were taken

Chronology—can be useful to get things in context

Final check with diary and notes. Are the details of dates and times given in the report accurate?

Does the report refer to quoted comments from any interviews? If so, is there a contemporaneous note, and is the report giving an accurate account of what the notes record?

If the report is based on information provided by others does the report make clear the nature of the information given, its source, the weight given to it, and the extent to which it has been relied on? Is there authority for disclosure of sources of information?

Does the report make clear the basis on which opinion is given and conclusions are drawn?

Has jargon been avoided?

Where technical terminology is unavoidable, is it also explained in clear terms?

Is the thinking process in the report clear and well reasoned?

Have all possible alternatives—for example, of diagnosis, treatment, assessment—been explored and evaluated, and is this made clear in the report?

Are there specific legal requirements for this case? Have they been met?

Are there specific legal requirements of format or content for this court report? Are they all fulfilled?

List of exhibits referred to in the report . . . and are they attached?

List of references cited, authorities quoted, or any other work relied on in the report; copies, if appropriate, attached as exhibits, or will they be available for use in court?

Police reports

In some cases of child abuse the police will ask for a report in the form of a witness statement. This needs to be on a police reporting form, which is available from either the local police station or the police officer who has asked for the report. Police officers like to come with their notebooks and write the report themselves and then present it to the doctor to sign. Many doctors do not like this because they find that the report they are asked to sign is written in language that they would not use ("I proceeded to the ward where I ascertained that the minor was in bed and commenced my investigation") or which does not quite reflect the opinion that they want to give (and would give if writing it themselves). Therefore most doctors prefer to write their own police report in the approved format and send it to the police station. Sending the report by post allows more time for necessary thought and preparation. A hastily written report may be harmful to the case and also to the reputation of the expert. Under no circumstances should a doctor give in to pressure from the police or any other agency to prepare a report too hastily. The police officers will make it clear which areas of information they want in the report. Police reports are usually much briefer than the lengthy medical report that may be required for court hearings.

Writing a report for the police does not necessarily mean that a prosecution will follow. Once the police have completed their investigation into alleged criminal offences the file is submitted to the Crown Prosecution Service for consideration of the evidence and for legal advice. When the evidence is sufficient the Crown Prosecution Service will conduct the case on behalf of the police.

The Director of Public Prosecutions has a different function. When certain serious criminal offences are suspected the director has the power to initiate an investigation into the matter and to authorise prosecution in the public interest.

Content of reports

● Do not give the child's address or any information that would identify foster carers or adoptive parents unless first cleared with the court or the instructing advocate.

● At the start give your full name, current position, and medical qualifications. Follow that with some indication of previous relevant experience—for example, "I have been a principal in general practice for 12 years" or "I am a paediatric registrar who has worked with children for five years". If you have had particular training or experience of child abuse mention its extent; if you have published research work on the subject say so.

● Make clear the nature of your interest in the case in terms of how you came to encounter the child and how long you have been concerned with the case and in what capacity. State the extent of your knowledge of the case in terms of correspondence and discussion with colleagues and the nature of the documents and reports that you have seen. Sometimes many hospital records and documents will have been studied, in which case a statement such as "I have studied the case notes and relevant documents" is sufficient.

• State the extent of your contact with the child—for example, "I examined the child in my outpatient clinic and discussed the problems with the parents. The consultation lasted 50 minutes" or "I assessed the child every month during the following year, each assessment lasting about 15 minutes".

• Summarise the case, being careful to amplify any medical jargon as the report will be read by many non-medical people and will probably be seen by the child's parents. Terms such as petechiae or apnoea need explanation. When relating the clinical history write it down chronologically and in addition to the date make clear the child's age at each incident.

• Clinical findings follow the history and should be set out in an ordered fashion. A diagram or photograph may be added to supplement the description. When the pattern of injury is typical—for example, finger marks showing a firm grip on a child or slap marks—an explanation of how and why that pattern is recognisable is helpful to lay people. Though the main findings may relate to a particular injury or to just one part of the body, always include a general appraisal of the child, including his or her height and weight (and their centile value) and a note on the child's developmental abilities. This should be followed by a note of the child's behaviour during the consultation or at any other times that you have observed the child with the parents or elsewhere.

• The conclusion or opinion should be clear but not too dogmatic. The court wants to know your opinion and if possible to evaluate it. Remarks such as "the findings are compatible with" can be extraordinarily unhelpful, and you should try to give an indicator of likelihood in terms of probability. State the reasons for your opinion in the report and be prepared to discuss them subsequently. Any confirmatory pathological or radiographical findings should be reported, explained, and interpreted.

• When providing an expert medical opinion in a statement for court, ensure that all known relevant reasons leading to the conclusion and opinions given are included in the original statement and clearly set out. If additional facts or reasons come to light after that statement is filed the court may give leave to file an additional statement. The courts may refuse to admit evidence of matters not contained in a statement filed with the court, since the other parties will not have had a chance to consider or refute whatever is being postulated.

• If you have seen a statement from another party that contradicts your opinion finish your statement by making clear which of your findings are consistent with the contradictory statement and which are not, making any relevant comments arising from those contradictions.

• Expert witnesses have additional roles. The duty of the expert may include an explanation of child development, child behaviour, and the effect of adverse factors such as abuse on the child. Thus the expert is drawing attention to the particular needs of the child for the benefit of those who have less experience with children. The expert witness may sit through the hearing to advise upon the different evidence presented. He or she may also be asked before the hearing to assess all the evidence and interview the family in order to present an authoritative opinion at the hearing.

Access to records and reports

The Access to Health Records Act 1990 came into force in 1991, giving rights to individuals in relation to non-computerised records held by health professionals about their physical or mental health. Computerised records are already covered by the Data Protection Act 1984.

The Access to Medical Reports Act 1988 gives qualified rights of access for individuals to medical reports prepared about them for employment or insurance purposes.

Further reading

Black D, Wolkind S, Hendriks JH. *Child psychiatry and the law.* London: Royal College of Psychiatrists, 1989.
Carson D. *Professionals and the courts.* Birmingham: Venture Press, 1990.
Gee DJ, Mason KJ. *The courts and the doctor.* Oxford Medical Publications, 1990.
Mitchels B, Prince A. *The Children Act and Medical Practice.* Family Law. Oxford: Jordan & Sons Ltd, 1992.

ABOUT COURTS

Barbara Mitchels, Roy Meadow

Even a fool can ask a question that an expert cannot answer.

DR JOHNSON

There are two types of court cases: criminal proceedings, in which a person is accused of an offence and is called on to answer the charge, either by admitting it, or by putting forward a defence; and civil proceedings, in which one person makes a claim against another for financial compensation or a judicial remedy, or both, such as an injunction, for an action which has caused some kind of damage. Family law is a subdivision of the civil law, in which remedies are sought for problems which arise within domestic life, including divorce, domestic injunctions, issues of maintenance of partners and children, and child care and protection. The Children Act 1989 defines "family proceedings" within which certain remedies are available, see the previous chapter *Child Care Law*

Evidence may be required from doctors in various different courts. The commonest will be child protection proceedings under the Children Act 1989. Sometimes the doctor will be a witness in the criminal prosecution of the alleged offender and, occasionally, in civil proceedings to resolve domestic issues arising from the incident—for example, an injunction or an action for damages or compensation, or both. Less than 3% of all child protection referrals result in a civil court hearing, and less than 0·5% lead to the prosecution of perpetrators.

The criminal and civil justice systems operate differently. In criminal cases, because a person's reputation and liberty may be at stake if they are convicted, the rules of evidence are strict, and it is the task of the prosecution to prove the case against the accused "beyond reasonable doubt". The court requires the "best evidence" and so will not permit certain types of evidence in hearing the case. The civil courts have a less strict standard of proof, the "balance of probabilities", in which the court has to be satisfied that the facts alleged are "more likely than not" to have occurred. In cases of child abuse, the more serious the allegations made the greater is the degree of proof required to establish the facts alleged.

There is a substantial difference in the approach of criminal and civil family proceedings. In criminal proceedings, which are adversarial, the objective is to ensure that the accused has a fair trial. Certain evidence is therefore excluded or restricted. In contrast, the paramount consideration for child protection proceedings under the Children Act 1989 is the welfare of the child, and so all relevant evidence should be put before the court to enable the court to make an informed decision in the child's best interests. Parents may have medical or psychiatric problems which affect their potential parenting ability. Recent case law now requires parties to disclose to the court and the other parties all medical and psychiatric reports, favourable or not. There are also provisions within the Children Act to encourage frank admission of child abuse in the proceedings, giving immunity from prosecution founded on such admissions. The guardian *ad litem* appointed to advise the court in child protection cases has access to all social work records. The guardian has no automatic right of access to medical records but may see those of a party with their consent and those of the child with appropriate consent or leave of the court. Note that any documents seen and mentioned in the guardian's report then become potentially admissible in evidence under the Children Act.

In both criminal and civil cases witnesses may be ordered to attend court by subpoena and to bring documents, including medical records (subpoena duces tecum). To avoid inconvenience let the lawyers or the court know in advance which dates to avoid when listing the case.

About courts

The Royal Courts of Justice in the Strand, London.

Criminal prosecutions

Criminal prosecution of adults commences in the *magistrates' court*. Criminal cases against young people under 18 commence in the *youth courts*. Serious criminal cases (including trials of young people in certain circumstances) will be committed to the crown court for trial. In the magistrates' court, the case is heard by three lay magistrates or a single, legally qualified, stipendiary magistrate, sometimes accompanied by a lay magistrate. Lay magistrates receive any necessary legal advice or guidance from the clerk to the court, who sits in front of them during the hearing and also takes notes of the evidence. A court usher is responsible for the smooth running of the case, noting who is present, locating witnesses who have disappeared to the cafeteria, and generally assisting the court.

In the *crown court* the case is heard by a judge sitting alone if the plea is guilty or by a judge and jury if the matter is contested. The judge has a clerk and a court usher to assist with administrative matters during the case. The crown court has a formal setting, with judge and advocates wearing wigs, gowns, and robes. The accused is likely to be in a dock, possibly guarded.

If an accused pleads guilty to the offence then, before sentencing, the magistrates or judge will hear evidence in mitigation, which may include medical and psychiatric assessments or recommendations. Evidence in criminal cases is by statement (see the previous chapter, *Medical Reports*) and oral evidence where required. If the matter is contested then evidence will be called in set order and the jury invited to bring in their verdict. The role of the judge is to advise the jury on matters of law, but issues of fact are for the jury to decide. Sentencing is a matter for the judge.

Appeals lie from the magistrates' court to the crown court (where appeals against conviction are retried) and also to the High Court by way of case stated (that is, without hearing the live evidence again). Appeals from the crown court lie to the Court of Appeal

(criminal division) and on a point of law of public importance to the House of Lords.

Child protection cases

The Children Act 1989 created one court, comprising three levels with similar powers so that cases may be transferred up or down the levels as appropriate to their gravity or complexity. Child protection cases may be brought in the magistrates' *family proceedings court*, in the *county court* care section, or the *High Court* family division. The hearings are "in camera", neither press nor visitors being given access. All the professionals involved have a common priority—the welfare of the child.

Appeals lie from the family proceedings court to the county court, and from the county court and High Court to the Court of Appeal (family division). Appeals on points of law of public importance may go to the House of Lords.

Evidence in these cases is by statement, filed with the court, and oral evidence when required by the court or parties to attend. Children Act statements are less formal than affidavits required in other civil cases and do not have to be sworn before a commissioner for oaths or court officer.

For civil or criminal proceedings statements may be agreed and then they may be read to the court. A witness need attend court only if requested to do so, usually because a statement needs clarification or is in some way disputed.

Court procedure

The procedure of the youth court, magistrates' court, and the crown court are similar. There will be seating allocated for advocates and parties, with separate seating or a witness box closer to the bench or judge for witnesses. There is likely to be security screening of those entering the court building, but this is usually compensated for by reasonable canteen facilities to offset the seemingly interminable waiting for cases to start. Magistrates' courts often have tea and coffee facilities open only for a limited time.

When you arrive at court the case will be listed by name and number in the public area. The usher needs to know the names of all participating in the case as they arrive and to know where to find witnesses when required. There are usually payphones in the public areas and in the advocates' rooms. To save embarrassment, switch off pagers and mobiles before entering the courtroom.

Entry into the courtroom can make important impressions. Dress soberly and unobtrusively, and try to be calm and unhurried. Try not to go into the witness box laden with coat, umbrella, bags, and shopping bought on the way to court. Have notes readily accessible, with markers on essential topics for easy referral, and know where to find necessary information. Use a ring binder that won't come apart if dropped. Be aware that the judge or others may ask to see the notes.

Rules of evidence

Ordinary witnesses may give evidence only of fact. Expert witnesses may also give their opinion. The court decides who is an expert witness. Qualifications and experience should be cited in a report for court (see the previous chapter *Medical Reports*).

In criminal cases, because the burden of proof is high, the court wants the "best evidence" possible, and therefore the rules about admissible evidence are strict. One of the most difficult rules is that concerning "hearsay", which is disallowed. Witnesses can tell the court only what they experienced for

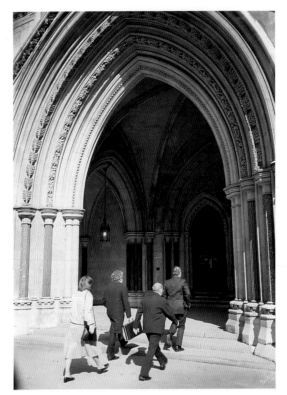

Layout of family proceedings court

Magistrates' bench	
| Chair |	Witness box

Court clerk

Guardian *ad litem*

Solicitor for child

Child (if old enough to attend court)

Local authority solicitor

Social worker

Expert witness

| Advocate for parent | Parent | Advocate for parent | Parent |

Order of evidence in contested cases

Criminal cases
- Parties introduced to the court
- Prosecution opens case
- Prosecution witnesses
- Defence witnesses
- Closing speech(es) for defence
- Judge sums up
- Jury/magistrates retire for decision

Child protection proceedings
- Parties introduced to court
- Applicant (usually local authority) opens case
- Applicant's witnesses
- Respondent's witnesses
- Child's evidence (if any)
- Guardian *ad litem*'s evidence
- Respondents closing speech
- Guardian *ad litem*'s closing speech
- Court retires for decison

Procedure for each witness
- Evidence in chief
- Cross examination
- Re-examination
- Court (magistrate/judge) questions witness

---

themselves not what others told them to prove the matters stated—for example, a child's examination record might note "John said while I examined him on March 7 1996 'Uncle Sid put his willie in my bum and it hurt'". This statement by the child would not be admissible in evidence at Sid's trial for a criminal sexual offence to prove the fact of penetration. It would be admitted only to prove that John was alive and well on March 4, capable of speaking, and that he spoke to the doctor during the examination. Medical evidence could report the examination results, which may include anal fissures, therefore corroborating the child's evidence. John would have to tell the court himself what Uncle Sid did. Video links are available in specified circumstances for young witnesses as an alternative to giving evidence in chief, but young witnesses still have to be available for cross examination, and this can be a distressing and potentially abusive experience for children and vulnerable adults. Attempts by advocates to discredit young vulnerable witnesses in adversarial proceedings are potentially emotionally abusive, and it is hoped that further legal protection will be forthcoming for vulnerable witnesses.

In contrast, because the ethos of family proceedings is to have before the court all possible relevant evidence to serve the interests of the child, in civil cases concerning the "upbringing, maintenance or welfare of a child" which includes child protection, the hearsay rule does not apply, and this statement could (and should) be cited by the witness. The court will decide what weight to give the evidence before it.

- Notes should be the originals, with any alterations and amendments clearly marked, dated, and signed. Be prepared to explain the

alteration. Notes from other colleagues may be included if part of a continuous medical record
• *x* ray pictures and photographs may be produced as exhibits and duly validated and identified by their maker, or, if they form part of medical records, they may be produced by the responsible health practitioner
• Samples and specimens may be produced as exhibits and duly identified by the person responsible for taking them or by the health practitioner. The Police and Criminal Evidence Act 1984 governs the taking of intimate samples from suspects in custody
• Computer print outs may be produced, provided properly verified
• Research findings, references, etc, may be used in court, but be prepared for cross examination by an advocate who may question the research sampling methods, hypotheses, aims, and evaluations, so know any work cited really well and bring a few copies to court in case the judge asks to see it.

Witnesses are not the property of any party in a case. Experts may wish to confer with each other, and it is courteous to do so in the presence of their respective instructing advocates, or at least with their knowledge. Experts should be independent and demonstrate this by non-partisan behaviour. It is wise to consult the advocate about any request to confer with any other party or witness. The court does not permit discussion by anyone with a witness when they are still giving evidence and there is an adjournment—for example, for lunch.

Ordinary witnesses have to wait outside the courtroom to prevent them being influenced by what others say. Expert witnesses are permitted to hear all the evidence to formulate an opinion on the basis of all available information. Sit near the instructing advocate if possible—they may need an expert's assistance as the case progresses. As a matter of courtesy, silence is observed in the court—audible asides or critical comment is unprofessional. If it is necessary to communicate urgently with the advocate, options are to pass a note or whisper if the comment is short, and if a longer consultation proves necessary, the advocate can seek a short adjournment.

It is traditional to stand for the entrance and exit of the magistrates or judge and to incline the head in deferential greeting as they enter. In the witness box, after the oath or affirmation, remain standing to give evidence until invited to sit. Behave with dignity, not pomposity, being courteous rather than ingratiating. It is dangerous to venture opinions on topics without the ability to justify them. Occasionally, in criminal trials, witnesses have to tolerate simulated anger, sarcasm, and obtuseness from advocates, and it is also tempting to respond in kind with a show of skill; resist the urge. When under attack, patient and calm response directed to the judge or bench pays dividends. Advocates ask questions which seem to be the result of relevant research but may well be just provocative ammunition. Treat this like a viva in an examination, and take such questions calmly, take time to consider the reply, then reply to the question asked, preferably without adding further unsolicited information, unless it is relevant and vital to the case.

Speak clearly and slowly enough for the judge and others to take their notes of points they need to record. Do not rush evidence, take time to think before answering questions. Be prepared to refer to your notes or medical records before answering. Be accurate and concise. If the answer is not known, say so. Direct replies to questions to the magistrates or the judge, rather than the advocate. It is then harder for an advocate to interrupt a witness in mid-flow with a different question to avoid the witness saying their next sentence, a subtle cross examination technique often used. If interrupted before you have said all you want, quietly and firmly return to the unfinished sentence first before answering the next question.

Expert witnesses have additional roles. The duty of the expert may include explaining child development, child behaviour, and the effect of adverse factors such as abuse on a child. Thus the expert is drawing attention to the particular needs of the child for the benefit of those who have less experience with children.

If it is necessary to leave after giving evidence, ask the court's consent to be released. Expenses of travel, accommodation,

---

Forms of address in court

• **My Lord or My Lady**: High Court judges or any deputy sitting as a High Court judge; and all judges sitting at the Central Criminal Court (the "Old Bailey")

• **Your Honour**: all circuit or district judges sitting in the crown court or the county court; and most other judges in the Commonwealth or United States

• **Sir** or **Madam**, or less commonly now, **Your Worship**: magistrates

It is customary to stand and bow the head to magistrates or judges when they enter or leave the courtroom. Similarly, when you enter or leave a court that is in session a modest bow to the bench or judge is appropriate.

and time spent in travelling and at court should be paid by the party calling the witness, agreed in advance, if necessary authorised by the legal aid board, and confirmed in writing to the witness by the instructing solicitor. The BMA produces a leaflet (No 33) giving guidelines for members on legal fees and allowances.

Try to make a good exit, picking up notes efficiently, and leaving with dignity. Bring a diary; if the case is adjourned it is helpful to know those dates to avoid for future hearings. Courts are usually considerate of doctors' clinical commitments and make every effort to assist by calling evidence at times suitable for the witness.

Anyone interested in sharing expertise among the legal, scientific, and medical professions may wish to contact the membership secretaries of the following associations:

Forensic Science Society, Clarke House, 18A Mount Parade, Harrogate, North Yorkshire HG1 1BX (tel 01423 506068).
British Academy of Forensic Sciences, The Secretariat, Department of Anaesthesia, The London Hospital Royal, London E1 2AD (tel 0171 377 7076).
Medico-Legal Society, Miss E Pygott, c/o Barlow Lyde & Gilbert, Beaufort House, 15 St Botolph Street, London EC3A 7NJ (tel 0171 247 2277).

ABUSE: THE EXPERIENCE

Within every type of child abuse there is a spectrum of severity. The severity depends not only on the duration, intensity, and context of the abuse but also on the way in which the family and the professionals deal with it.

The first set of abstracts have been compiled by Sylvia Fraser from her book in which she tells a story which is common. For many years she thought that she was an ordinary person until incestuous memories returned, at which stage she feared she was a freak. Her recognition that sexual abuse within the family is common was, in a strange way, a comfort; she realised that she was still an ordinary person. She makes clear that the denial in her family was a reflection of the denial in the society that bred us all.

Towards the other end of the spectrum is someone else's experience, recounted with clarity and intensity 50 years after it happened—on the beach.—RM

My Father's House—Sylvia Fraser

My father's house was a three storey, frame building on a shady street in Hamilton, Ontario. Though our family found it hard to grow grass because of maple roots, our lawn was always neatly trimmed, our leaves raked, and our snow shovelled. No one drank in my father's house, no one smoked, and no one took the Lord's name in vain. Though my father worked on shifts at the Steel Company of Canada, he always wore a white shirt, navy suit, and tie to his job as a steel inspector— trace memory of a family that had once been prosperous. I was born into my father's house on March 8, 1935 . . . .

I sit on my daddy's lap playing tick tack toe under the glare of a fringed and faded lamp. I have the Xs, he has the Os. I get three across: "I'm the winner!"

There's not much room on my daddy's lap because of his big tummy, held up by a black belt. His tummy feels warm against my cheek. The buttons on his shirt are pearly in the light. I run my fingers down them singing: "Tinker, tailor, soldier, sailor".

My sister, Helen, who is four years older, says: "When you run out of buttons that's the man you have to marry!"

Twice every Sunday my family drives to St James's United Church in my daddy's secondhand Ford-with-a-running-board. I wear white stockings and carry my Dionne Quintuplet handkerchief with a nickel tied in one corner. That is for the collection. My father and three other gentlemen carry the silver plates tramp tramp tramp up to the altar where Reverend Thwaite blesses them, "Thank you, Fatherrr, forrr yourrr bountiful blessings." He means God.

We drive home past the statue of Queen Victoria with a bird's nest on her head and the 16 storey Pigott building, which I know to be the tallest in the world, with my daddy honking every time we get stuck behind a belt-line streetcar. At the foot of Wentworth Street he points to a pile of weathered boards on the side of the Mountain. "That's where the old incline used to run".

I know by now he means a cable car that once ran on a track to the top. Pressing my face against the glass, I stare at this heap of boards, buried in undergrowth. Try as I do, I can make no connection between what I see and the wonder in my daddy's voice. Yet his reverence for things that once were and can never be again inspires my favourite name, the one I use to baptise my oldest and dearest friend: Teddybear Umcline.

Down down down the stairs I go, dragging Teddy Umcline by one ear. My daddy sits framed in his doorway in trousers and undershirt. As I scuff my running shoe over the brass strip marking the threshold, he puts out his black shoe, which he has trouble reaching because of his tummy. I get down on my hands and knees to tie his lace. My daddy smells of Lifebuoy soap. He rubs his face against mine. That's a whisker rub. "You're tickling me!"

My daddy plays with my blond hair. "I had curls like that when I was your age". He plays with my belly button and jiggles pennies in his pocket. My daddy squeezes my legs between his knees. I count my pennies, already imagining them to be black balls and red liquorice from the Candy Factory. The breeze through the window smells of lilacs. It blows the curtains inward like Rapunzel's golden hair, giving me goose bumps.

My daddy and I share secrets.

My mother sprinkles my father's starched white shirts with water from a vinegar bottle. She is reciting a story I know ends with a mouse piping: "Gee whillikers, an owl's egg!" I rock on a hamper of freshly washed clothes, pretending to listen but really worrying if I'll be smart in school.

My grade one teacher is Miss Warner, who is like a barrel with no neck and no waist. Arlene Goodfellow says once when Miss Warner was giving the strap her pants fell down to her ankles!

I am the first to learn all the voices of the vowels and to read the adventures of Dick and Jane and Spot and Puff through to the end. In the cloakroom I teach the other kids to tie their shoelaces in a double bow just like my daddy taught me.

My daddy plays with my belly button, my daddy plays with my toes as he did when I was little: "This little piggy, that little piggy . . . ." Now I lie on my daddy's bed, face buried in his feather pillow. I shiver, because the window is open, the lace curtains are blowing, and I haven't any clothes on. My daddy lies beside me in his shorts and undershirt, smelling of talcum. He rubs against me, still hot and wet from his bath. My daddy breathes very loudly, the way he does when he snores, and his belly heaves like the sunfish I saw on the beach at Van Wagners. Something hard pushes up against me, then between my legs and under my belly. It bursts all over me in a sticky stream. I hold my breath, feeling sick like when you spin on a piano stool till the seat falls off. I'm afraid to complain because daddy won't love me won't love me love me.

I cry when my mother puts me to bed. I didn't used to be afraid of the dark but now I know that demons and monsters hide in the cubbyholes by my bed. I'm afraid one will jump out at me, and rub dirty dirty up against me with its wet-ums sticking out. I beg my mother to stay with me but she says, "Such a fuss!"

I have a scary night. My pillow tries to smother me with its dead feathers. When I wake up I am facedown in vomit. It smells like chicken guts.

Desperation makes me bold. At last I say the won't-love-me words: "I'm going to tell my mummy on you!"

My father replaces bribes with threats. "If you do, you'll have to give me back all your toys".

I tote up my losses: my Blondie and Dagwood cutouts, my fairytale colouring book, my crayons! "My mummy gave those things to me. They're mine".

"I paid for them. Everything in this house belongs to me. If you don't behave I've a good mind to throw them into the furnace".

I think of my beloved Teddy Umcline, his one good eye melting in the flames. "I don't care! I don't care! I don't care!"

"Shut up! What will the neighbours think? If you don't shut up I'll . . . I'll . . . send you to the place where all bad children go. An orphanage where they lock up bad children

whose parents don't want them any more."

"My mother won't let you!"

"Your mother will do what I say. Then you'll be spanked every night and get only bread and water."

That shuts me up for quite a while, but eventually I dare to see this, too, as a game for which there is an answer: "I don't care. I'll run away!"

My father needs a permanent seal for my lips, one that will murder all defiance. "If you say once more that you're going to tell I'm sending that cat of yours to the pound for gassing!"

"I'll . . . I'll . . . I'll . . ."

The air swooshes out of me as if I have been punched. My heart is broken. My resistance is broken. Smoky's life is in my hands. This is no longer a game, however desperate. Our bargain is sealed in blood.

I lie on my stomach on the living room rug, colouring in my fairytale book. I colour the hair of all the princesses with my yellow crayon—Cinderella and Sleeping Beauty and Rapunzel.

My father sits in his fetch-me chair working a crossword puzzle. His pencil snaps. He grunts: "Fetch me a paring knife."

I colour Cinderella's eyes blue, then turn the page to Sleeping Beauty.

"I'm talking to you!"

I colour Sleeping Beauty's eyes blue.

The floor trembles under my tummy. "Fetch me a paring knife."

I shuffle to the kitchen, s-t-r-e-t-ching the seconds like a rubber band, enjoying the terrible tension while wondering when it will snap. I hand my father the knife with the blade toward him, then return to my spot on the floor. With a black crayon, I outline the naked bodies of Cinderella and Sleeping Beauty and Rapunzel, right through their clothes, repeating ME ME ME. Then MINE MINE MINE.

Staring at my father's black boot, I boldly form the thought: I hate you . . . God does not strike me dead. I do not turn to stone. I repeat: hate hate hate hate hate, enjoying the sharp taste of the word like a lozenge in my mouth.

My arms stick to my sides, my legs dangle like worms as my daddy forces me back against his bed. I love my daddy. I hate my daddy. Love hate love hate. Daddy won't love me love me hate hate hate. I'm afraid to strike him with my fists. I'm afraid to tell my mummy. I know she loves Helen because she is good, but she doesn't like me because I am dirty dirty. Guilt fear guilt fear fear dirty dirty fear fear fear fear fear fear.

One day I can stand it no longer. I unscrew my head from my body as if it is the lid of a pickle jar. From now on there will be two of me—a child who knows, and a child who dares not know any longer. She will be my daddy's sexual accomplice. Though we will share the same body, I will not know of her existence. I will not experience, or remember, anything she does with daddy, and my loss of memory will be retroactive. I will not remember my daddy ever touching me sexually. I will not remember ever seeing my daddy naked. I will not remember my daddy ever seeing me naked. In future whenever my daddy approaches me sexually I will turn into my other self, and afterwards I will not remember anything that happened. This memory block will last 40 years.

On the Beach and Afterwards

When the midday meal was over my brother and I walked along the beach in front of our house. This was 50 years ago. I was 8 and my brother 7 years old. After walking a quarter of a mile we saw a man sitting by himself at the foot of the beach retaining wall in an angle where steps led down to the sand from the road. The beach was part of a friendly suburban community where people usually greeted each other whether they knew them or not. So we said hello to this pleasant stranger who gave us a sweet. After some talk he invited us to tickle his chest and abdomen with one of the long pine needles which lay in the sand. I noticed that he didn't have swimming trunks on and had covered his lower abdomen and thighs with a towel. When my brother asked about this he said that he belonged to a group which liked to bathe without any clothing. Soon he moved the towel aside and asked for the pine needles to be brought lower until they stroked his penis. Then he asked where we could go so that we could not be seen.

A few yards away the Home Guard had built a slit trench some eight feet long and six feet deep with boarded sides to stop subsidence, part of the coastal defences. We went over to it and climbed down, concealed from passersby.

In the trench he dropped the towel and asked me to take hold of his now erect penis and rub it. This I did with my brother looking on. He said, "Do it harder," and then, "Do it faster". After a short time white fluid came out and splashed on to the floor of the trench. He then put on his bathing trunks, climbed out, and returned to the beach with us and made us promise not to tell what had happened.

We were excited and puzzled by this novel event and described it to my mother when we got home. She made us soak our hands in disinfectant and said we must not tell my father, but she did so. He questioned us, became silent with a grim look around his mouth as he did when angry, and insisted we go at once and search the beach. When I asked "Why?" he said he was going to thrash the man, adding we were lucky that he had not put his penis up our backsides. My father and I walked the beach without finding the man and then went to the police, which my mother opposed. There we told our story to the village policeman, a dull man with prominent front teeth who wrote it down in long hand in pencil.

My next memory is of walking along a line of men and pointing out the man. Then followed a magistrates' court hearing in a small room when I had to tell the story again, this time in front of the man. I could not look at him. We had promised not to tell anyone and had broken the promise. Then there was a wait of some months until the trial.

For the trial we had the afternoon off school. My father took us to the High Court waiting room and left us alone and we had a fight. My brother and I often had fights which I usually won because I was bigger and more aggressive. He hit me hard on the nose and it would not stop bleeding. My appearance in court had to be delayed while attempts were made to stop the bleeding with a cold sponge to my forehead and a key dropped down my back. Then when the bleeding stopped I heard my name being called repeatedly in the way it is in films of courtroom dramas. I was conducted to the courtroom and stood in the witness stand. A man in black in the centre of the room asked my name and then said, "Do you see the accused here?" I replied, "What does accused mean?" Some discussion followed and I was told, "It means the man who is said to have done these things". I looked around the courtroom inspecting I imagine reporters, the public, the jury, the lawyers, and the judge and began to think he was not there. Then I saw him, in the centre of the court surrounded with a rail, pointed, and said, "There he is". I was asked to say what had happened on the beach and then questioned. This was the fifth or sixth time I had gone through the story in an official setting. One question used the name of a different beach as the site of the offence, which I corrected. I wondered subsequently if the wrong name was a test of my lying. My brother then gave evidence and my father took us home.

That in a way was the end of the affair for me, but in another way it was the beginning of a lifelong memory, which from time to time I think through or discuss with a confidant.

In writing this account I have tried to decide what harm I came to as a result of the sexual experience, corruption as the judge stated when sentencing. I have concluded, with possible lack of insight, no harm of consequence. A benefit has been some limited understanding of sexual contact between an adult and child. But the trial, the preparation for it, and the aftermath did cause much worry and helped reinforce the memory so that I am able to write this piece confident in the accuracy of the facts and emotions recalled.

My brother and I shared a bedroom and talked a lot about what had happened. We were worried for some months about the man escaping and coming to look for us to kill or harm us. I have never been aware of feeling ashamed or stigmatised, but did elect to publish this account unsigned. The absence of a sense of shame or stigma resulted partly from the offender being nice to us, partly from my parents, who never made us feel guilty, and partly from the authorities' approach. They tried to ascertain the facts without making a fuss and indirectly conveyed to us that we were not responsible for what had happened.

This absence of responsibility might not be entirely true for it could be said that I colluded to some extent both with the man and with the authorities. My emotion at the time of the act was of intense curiosity and excitement. My brother remembers the same. We had never seen a naked adult man or an erect adult penis. The man had not forced us into stimulating him and we could have left at any time without risk of violence. Subsequently it was probably satisfying to ally myself with the authorities in the pursuit of the wrongdoer with myself as the wronged child, the centre of attention.

The newspaper report of the trial says that verdicts of guilty were returned on eight charges of indecent assault on boys and one charge of committing an indecent act with intent to insult. The judge, awarding a sentence of 12 years' imprisonment, remarked on the corrupting influence on boys and a previous sentence of four years for the same offence. He declared that the man was an habitual criminal and a menace to the community. I do not know what happened to him. He would have been 58 years of age on release from prison after a full sentence.

The abstracts compiled by Sylvia Fraser are from her book, *My father's house—a memoir of incest and of healing* by permission of the publishers, Virago Press.

On the Beach and Afterwards was first published as an anonymous personal view in the *British Medical Journal* 23 November 1991.

INDEX

Index